Unforgettable Patients

Also by James Y Hung:

Finding Fat Lady's Shoe: A Memoir of Growing up in Hong Kong and Malaysia (2013)

FOB in Paradise: A Memoir (2014)

Silk Road on My Mind (2015)

Practical Ophthalmology: A Concise Manual for the Non-Ophthalmologist (2016)

The Chinese Language Demystified (2018)

Introduction to Tang Poetry (2019)

Sightless: A Novel (2019)

I Left My Heart in Malaya (2020)

Class of 1964 (2021)

Cambodia On My Mind (2021)

Samoa On My Mind (2022)

Available through Amazon in paperback and Kindle e-book. E-book also available through Barnes & Noble.

Finding Fat Lady's Shoe

An intensely reflective tale of a family uprooted by war, cast adrift onto a sea of uncertainty.—Kirkus Review

Dr. James Hung's life story echoes others that will probably never be written, and offers a fascinating perspective on Hong Kong's recent past that deserves to be widely read. [4 stars out of 5]—South China Morning Post

FOB in Paradise

Hung has written an absorbing and witty book. Dramatic, nuanced vignettes and vivid descriptions of people and places create a rich tapestry that shows the medical profession at its best and worst.
—Kirkus Review

Silk Road on My Mind

Hung is an endearing mix of benevolence, wryness, and curiosity....there is an appealing Marco Polo-ishness to his project: a boundless wonder for a society unlike his own, not for its differences but for the infinitely recognizable humanity at its center.—Kirkus Review

Practical Ophthalmology

More specialists should create guides of this caliber for nonspecialists. An indispensable ophthalmological volume for any general practitioner's office.—Kirkus Review (featured article 11/15)

The Chinese Language Demystified

An engrossing introduction to the riches of Chinese that should delight casual language mavens and more experienced speakers alike.—Kirkus Review (featured article 6/15)

Introduction to Tang Poetry

...will be accessible to novices and a rich resource for experts.... A compelling, detail-rich resource about Tang verse.—Kirkus Review (featured article 3/1)

Sightless: A Novel

An engaging tale about a singular friendship that gives voice to the struggles of the sightless.—Kirkus Review (featured article 2/15)

I Left My Heart in Malaya

With great tenderness, he recounts the beautiful simplicity of that stretch of his youth...—Kirkus Review

Class of 1964

Hung's prose is clean and leisurely. The book is valuable for the portrait it paints of Hong Kong in the 1960s—a melting pot of cultures, settling refugees, and immigrants from across the world that's fending off the looming menace of mainland China.

—Kirkus Review

Cambodia On My Mind

A sensitive, wide-ranging introduction to a diverse Southeast Asian nation grappling with its past.

... [Hung's] detailed vignettes, recalling his experiences and inquisitive conversations with everyone from doctors to "tuk tuk" drivers, paint a vibrant portrait of daily life, customs, foods, and challenges experienced throughout Cambodian society.—Kirkus Review

Samoa On My Mind

Hung is an amusing and straightforward narrator, but he doesn't shy away from discussing the heaviness of the medical workload for those working in the Samoan islands or corruption in the Samoan government. An immersive and expansive, yet highly personal, account of a compelling locale and its people.—Kirkus Review

Unforgettable Patients

James Y Hung MD

Unforgettable Patients

ISBN: 978-1-7353552-4-5 (James Y Hung)

Edited by Anne Correia

Contents

Author's Note

A RECENT SURVEY OF PHYSICIANS in the US showed that 9 out of 10 would not recommend the profession to anyone, especially their children. This is a sad state of affairs for a profession. I can understand the frustrations of many physicians now as they deal with more and more paperwork, rules and regulations. Many of them are simply burnt out.

I was lucky to have practiced medicine when I did. It was a kinder and gentler time. Physicians treated each other with respect and in most cases they even helped each other instead of viewing each other as competitors. There was no such a thing as advertising in our profession in those days.

I was more than happy to take care of other physicians and their families free of charge, and they could call on me anytime. Likewise, they were happy to take care of me and my family and I could call on them anytime. Most of us were happy to donate our time teaching residents and medical students. We never expected anything in return other than feeling that it was our turn to pay it back to society.

I'm grateful that I was able to get into medical school and become an eye surgeon. I cannot imagine having gone into another field. Being a doctor is part of my identity, my *raison d'être*. There's no other profession that would have allowed me to travel all over the world to help people. Unlike some other specialties, such as ob/gyn, an ophthalmologist faces no taboo in any country or culture.

One of the greatest satisfactions of being a physician is when you relieve your patient's pain or improve their life. Another is when you know your patient feels that you care.

Chapter 1

Baptism by Fire

IT WAS LIKE A WAR ZONE. Blood was everywhere. People were crying with pain. There had been a multiple vehicle wreck on Highway 99, the main north-south freeway in California.

It was mid-August of 1974 and I was about six weeks into my first rotation of an internship at the Valley Medical Center (VMC), the major trauma hospital between Los Angeles and San Francisco, and a teaching hospital affiliated with the University of California San Francisco Medical Center (UCSF).

VMC had residency programs in most specialties with the exception of orthopedics and neurosurgery. The orthopedic care was contracted to a four-member orthopedic group in town. They rotated at VMC, supervising the clinic and giving recommendations to the general surgery residents who ended up providing most of the care.

In medical school, I had been interested in orthopedics. My plan was to do an internship in California, then return to Omaha to do my orthopedics residency at the University of Nebraska Medical Center. In competitive specialties like orthopedics, first-year resident spots were usually given out two years in advance, while we were still in medical school, before we even knew where we were going to do our internship. In anticipation of this, I'd taken a one-month rotation in orthopedic surgery in medical school; but most of my experience was with office orthopedics, which consisted mostly of patients with low back pain or hip and knee problems.

The wreck on Highway 99 had brought in five seriously injured patients, and all the surgical residents were in surgery trying to save their lives. The less severely injured were being cared for by the interns.

As I'd been on the orthopedic rotation for almost six weeks, I had already seen a great deal of trauma. Dr. Rod Fast, a second-year surgical resident and the only surgical resident at the ER, was helping further evaluate some of the less severe injuries.

Doug—another intern—and I were to take care of all the orthopedic problems, while the residents of the Emergency Medicine Program helped triage the patients.

A truck driver involved in the accident had an obvious fracture on his right leg. The upper end of the fracture had punctured through the skin. The X-ray showed a displaced fracture of the lower tibia.

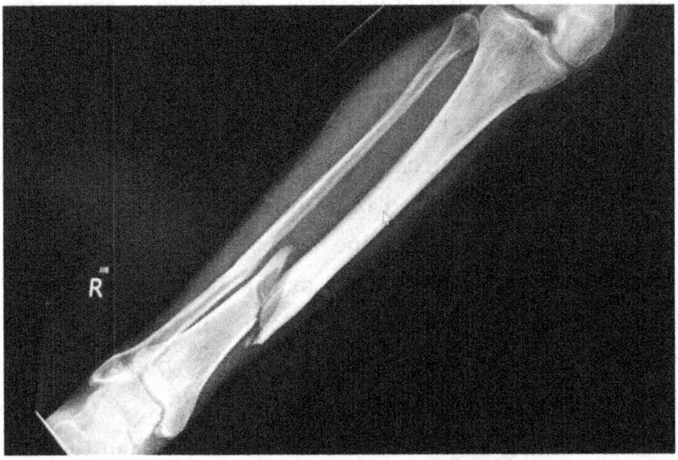

Fracture of the lower right tibia

The other bone, the smaller fibula, was intact. Luckily for this patient, screws (without a plate) would be able to reconnect the two ends of the tibia because the unbroken fibula provided stability.

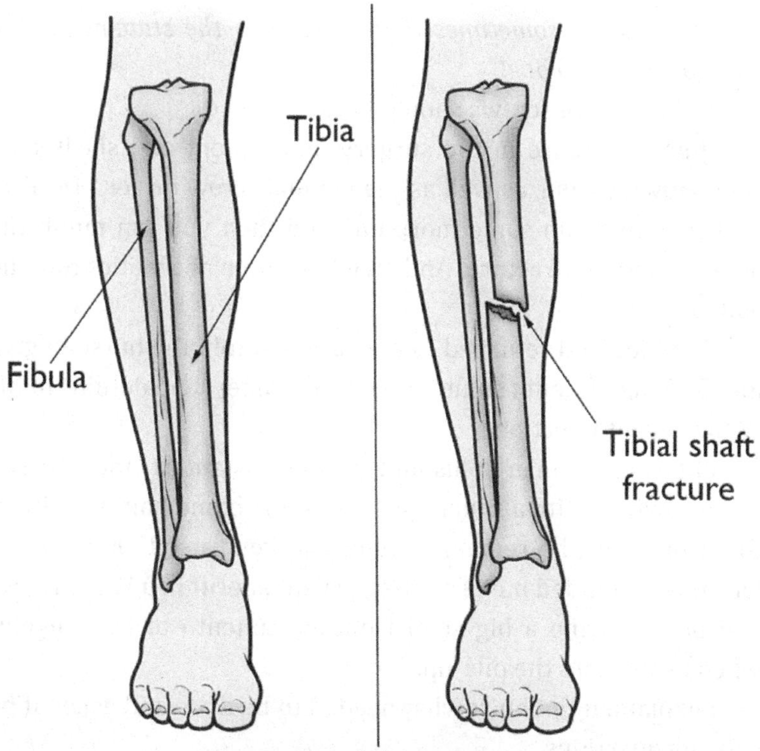

Anatomy of the lower leg

In this case, the patient would need a plate to join the two ends of the tibia because screws alone would not be able to affix the two ends of the fractured bone.

I found Dr. Fast, who was busy taking care of other surgical patients, and showed him the patient's X-ray and described the injury. To my surprise, he said, "Looks like it's one that you can fix. As you can see, you'll have to align the two ends of the tibia. Because it's not a clean fracture and the two ends aren't aligned, you need to put in some screws," Dr. Fast finished with a smile.

I'd seen it done before, but usually in an operating room. Since all the operating rooms were in use, Dr. Fast suggested that I do it in the minor surgery room at the ER.

In medicine, sometimes there's truth to the statement, "See one, do one, teach one!"

"What sort of screws should I use?" I asked.

"Just call Claire in the surgery department and she'll send some down to you, as well as the manual screw driver," Dr. Fast replied. "Give him some morphine and then you can numb the area around the fracture. And give him some antibiotics too," he added.

I nodded and returned to my patient. I told the nurse to give him 500 mg of Keflin solution (generic name: cephalothin) in his IV to prevent infection.

Chuck was a man in his mid-thirties, big and strong, dressed like a cowboy, with a square jaw and short blond hair. In spite of the broken leg, he remained quiet and kept a soft smile on his face that reminded me of a strong, silent sheriff in a Western. He had been driving a big semi from Sacramento to Los Angeles when he ran into the pile-up.

I explained to Chuck what needed to be done and asked if he had any questions.

"I'm feeling pretty good now, probably because of the morphine," Chuck commented. "Just do what you need to do. I have confidence in you. I like Japanese and Chinese doctors because I think they're smart and good with their hands."

His remark about Asian doctors surprised me. He had the look of an Okie—someone who had migrated from Oklahoma to California during the Dust Bowl and would generally be regarded as a redneck.

"Thanks Chuck. I appreciate your confidence," I responded.

In my rush to the hospital that day, I'd forgotten my glasses at home. So, I called my wife Mary and asked her to bring them, and in the meantime began formulating a plan for the procedure. A package was brought in to me by Marla, a highschool girl wearing the red and white candy stripe uniform for young volunteers. The sterile package consisted of two manual screwdrivers, six titanium screws and several hand instruments used in minor surgery such as needle holders, hemostats and scalpels.

As the tibia was easily palpable, just beneath the skin, I wouldn't need to do any dissection. An ER nurse was my assistant. She painted the skin around the fracture with Betadine solution and placed a few sterile green towels to isolate the operating field.

When Mary arrived with my glasses, she was astonished that I was about to put screws into this man's leg bone.

To my amazement, Chuck still had a smile on his face.

"It may be a little uncomfortable when I give you the Xylocaine to numb the area," I explained. "I think a little Valium would help."

"Sounds good," replied Chuck.

The nurse administered 5 mg of Valium in his IV, and soon I could see that Chuck's eyelids were barely open.

I infiltrated the Xylocaine solution around the wound and into the muscles, then enlarged the skin wound so I would have a better view of the two ends of the tibia.

Making sure Chuck wasn't feeling any of my manipulations, I connected the two ends of the fractured tibia. I then carefully placed three screws to secure the two ends. The reconnected tibia now looked straight. Finally, I closed the skin with several black silk sutures.

Before long, Chuck opened his eyes and was surprised to discover that I'd already finished. An orderly wheeled him to the X-ray department.

I was busy with another patient, so I asked the orderly to bring Chuck's film to the ER when it was ready. When I saw it, I was relieved that the two ends of Chuck's tibia came together very nicely and all the screws were securely placed in his bone.

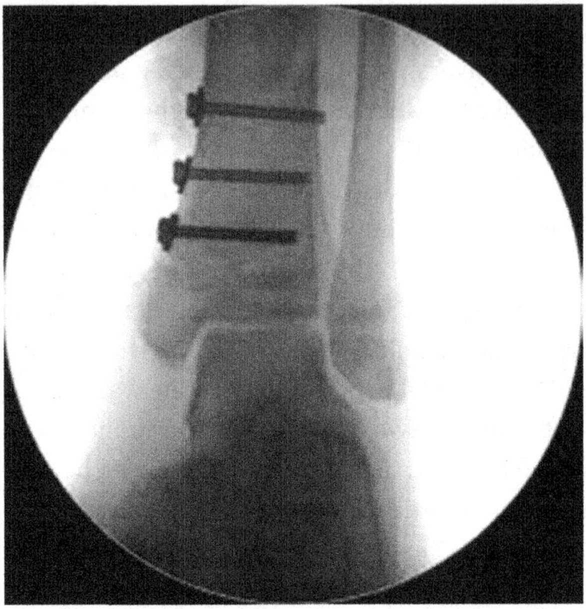

X-ray showing screws in the tibia

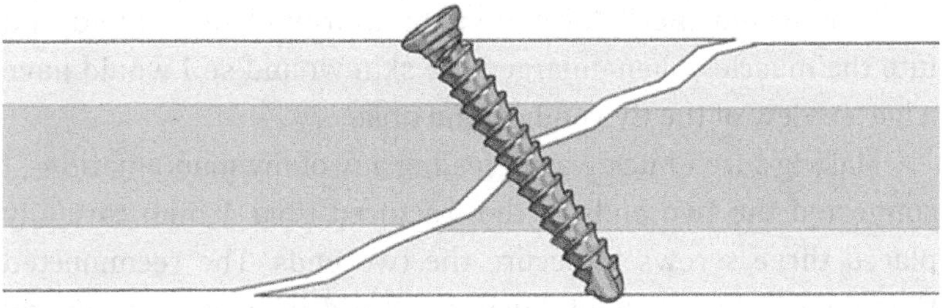

A titanium screw securing the two ends of the tibia

A technician in the ER put a cast on Chuck's leg from below the knee to his toes, and he was admitted to our service on the fifth-floor orthopedic ward to continue his IV antibiotics treatment as well as pain management.

Chuck never complained throughout the entire hospital stay and was followed in the outpatient clinic.

Soon I was finished with my orthopedic rotation and on to the dreaded four-month internal medicine rotation. Before I left the service, I asked Manuel, the cast technician in the clinic, to page me when Chuck returned for his follow-up.

Six weeks later, Chuck had his cast removed, and to my relief his leg was not crooked. He demonstrated the success of the surgery by walking around the clinic, showing no discomfort.

Thinking back to so many years ago, it was amazing that they allowed an intern to put screws in a patient's fractured leg. I don't think any hospital would let that happen now. If any complications developed, it would be difficult for the hospital to defend a lawsuit. Fortunately for me, and for Chuck, everything worked out well.

Chapter 2
Brain Surgery

IN MY LAST YEAR OF MEDICAL SCHOOL, I took another 4-week rotation in family practice at the University Hospital. The senior resident, Dr. Handley, was a 1970s hippie with a long, dark brown ponytail and a thick beard down to his sternum. He was a slight man, a little shorter than my five feet seven inches, and he wore gold wire-rimmed glasses. To me, he looked like a mountain man.

He was a free spirit, but he must have been an excellent student because he graduated from UCSF, one of the best medical schools in the country at the time. It took him seven years to graduate because he took three years off to work in Africa and the Middle East.

After his internship, he had to pay the US government back for his student loans and grants by working in a US Public Health Hospital for two years. These hospitals are usually located on Native American reservations. Dr. Handley was assigned to such a hospital in New Mexico, in the desert, on the Navajo Nation. The reservation had about 100,000 members of the Navajo tribe, and included a vast area of approximately 27,000 square miles.

He told me many scary stories about his time there, one of which was about a patient he saw with a collapsed lung. The X-ray machine wasn't working that day, so Dr. Handley had to depend on his statoscope to decide which side he should put the chest tube into. The side of the collapsed lung wouldn't have any breathing sounds coming from it.

He was petrified. If he put the chest tube on the wrong side, the patient would die.

He cried out with a sigh of relief when the patient's collapsed right lung was re-inflated, and he was no longer short of breath.

With a serious look on his face, he told me another story about another patient who wasn't so fortunate.

The hospital was at least five hours from the next town with a larger hospital, and the patient died in the ambulance on the way there to see a neurosurgeon, because Dr. Handley didn't know how to do a procedure called a burr hole.

He never forgave himself for that, knowing he could have saved the patient if he'd learned the procedure.

After hearing the story, I decided that if I had the chance, I would learn how to do it.

***

Burr Hole Surgery

The burr hole procedure is literally making a hole in the skull. The Incas were known to do this type of surgical procedure—known as trepanation—several thousand years ago, most likely to relieve the pressure in the brain, just as we do today.

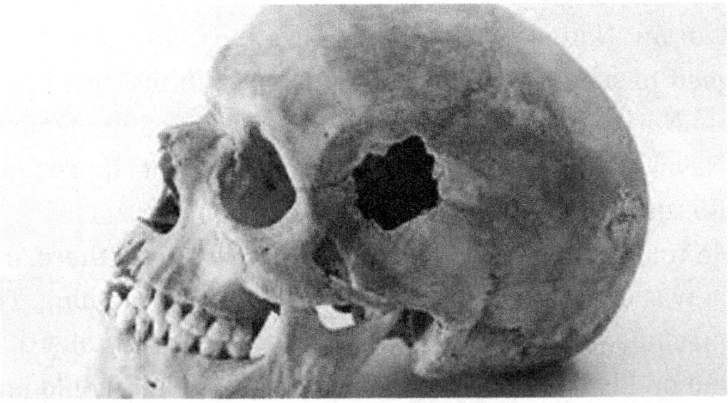

A 3000-year-old Inca skull showing a healed hole in the skull

Research on these skulls shows that trepanation was most frequently performed on men, possibly to treat injuries sustained in combat.

In Peru, about 800 prehistoric trepanned skulls have been recovered, well preserved thanks to the country's dry climate and high elevation. Researchers examining the skulls determined that if the edges of the hole showed significant signs of healing, the surgery was deemed successful; and skulls with ragged edges or no signs of healing likely meant that the patient hadn't survived the surgery or had died not long after.

***

During my internship, I had one month on the neurosurgical service.

The head of the neurosurgery department was a man from South Vietnam who had arrived in the country less than a year earlier. In Saigon, he was the head of the neurosurgery department of the largest medical school in South Vietnam. He had graduated from the same medical school and did his neurological surgery training in Paris, under some of the best-known neurosurgeons in France at the time. But the situation in South Vietnam was worsening and he and his family had decided to flee the country.

Dr. Tran was a little man who looked to be in his sixties. He had sparse gray hair on both sides and the back of his head. He was just over five feet tall and had bowed legs that were quite obvious. He explained to me that he had rickets caused by a Vitamin D deficiency when he was a baby because his family was so poor.

Unlike some of the neurosurgeons I knew, Dr. Tran was a friendly, somewhat reserved man who was easy to work with. The neurosurgeon I witnessed in medical school was a tyrant who actually threw surgical instruments at nurses and residents when things weren't going well. The medical students were too low on the ladder for him to be bothered with. He simply ignored us.

VMC was the only major trauma hospital between San Francisco and Los Angeles, so we saw a great deal of trauma.

One Friday night, a woman was brought into the ER by ambulance from the nearby town of Reedley, some 20 miles southeast of Fresno. Earlier in the day, she had fallen from her horse. Her family became concerned when her speech became slurred and she seemed confused.

Hayley Hutchins was a very attractive 20-year-old woman with shoulder-length caramel colored hair, still dressed in her riding clothes—a white shirt and long, tight dark blue pants.

When she was brought to the ER, she seemed confused, not knowing what month or year it was. She also had a balance problem and couldn't walk in a straight line. She said her head was hurting and she felt nauseated.

All her signs and symptoms pointed to pressure in her brain. The ER resident was concerned that she might have bleeding inside her brain and called the resident on the neurosurgical service. As VMC didn't have a neurosurgery residency, patients were taken care of by general surgery residents.

Soon, Dr. Newfeld, the senior surgical resident, and I arrived to evaluate the patient and Dr. Newfeld agreed with the ER resident that she might be bleeding inside her skull. X-rays of her head were performed immediately and confirmed the diagnosis of subdural hematoma.

In 1974, CT scans were just beginning to be used and they took a long time. As Hayley's condition was deteriorating rapidly, there was no time to wait for the technician to set up the CT machine. MRI wasn't yet invented.

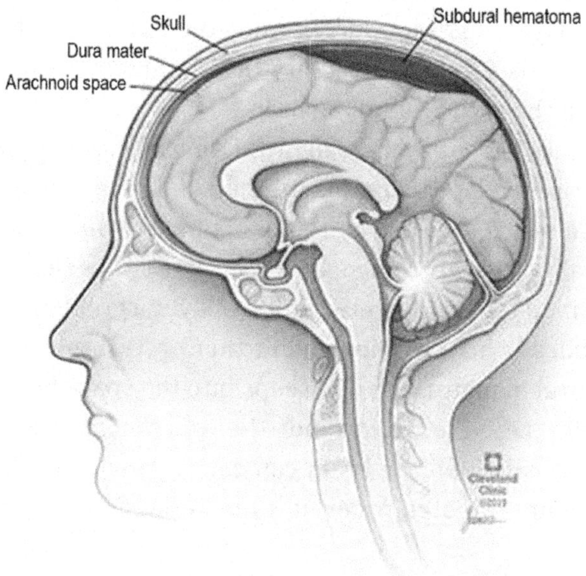

Subdural hematoma

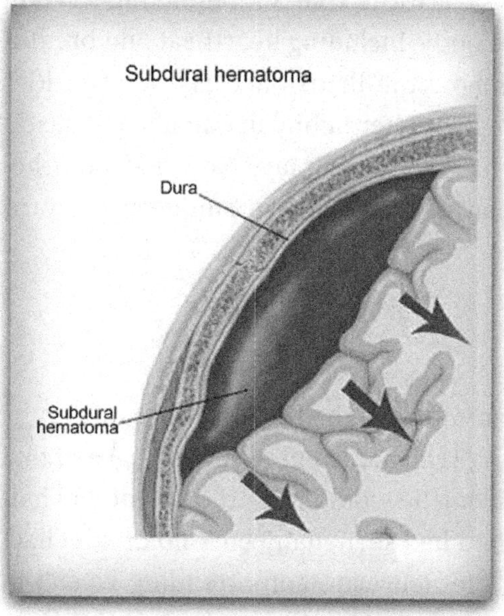

Pressure inside the skull causing damage to the brain

A subdural hematoma involves the buildup of blood between the protective layers of tissue surrounding the brain. The bleeding is frequently caused by a head injury that results in a blood vessel breaking in the area around the brain.

There are three layers, called the *meninges*, that cover the brain: the outer layer, just inside the skull, is a tough, fibrous membrane called the *dura mater*, or simply the *dura*; the middle layer is called the *arachnoid*; and the membrane closest to the brain is called the *pia*. In between each layer, cerebrospinal fluid fills the space to help cushion and further protect the brain.

In a subdural hematoma, blood seeps into the space between the two outer—i.e., the *dura* and the *arachnoid*—layers. The resulting pressure on the brain can cause damage to the tissue and can be life-threatening, even if the initial injury itself seems mild.

This is especially dangerous when the brainstem is being pushed downward by the pressure in the brain, as the brain stem serves a critical role in regulating certain involuntary actions of the body, including heartbeat and breathing.

This was how the British actress Natasha Richardson died. She was skiing with her family in Canada and sustained what the family thought was minor injury. She died a few hours later. Had she been seen at a hospital, a simple procedure would have saved her life.

***

Hayley was admitted to the ICU, awaiting surgery.

I called Dr. Tran at his home, and he agreed that surgery was necessary, saying he would be at the hospital in half an hour.

Dr. Newfeld had seen many burr holes, and had himself done a few when the neurosurgeon attending wasn't available. As a general surgeon in training, he really had little interest in doing more burr holes, and since he was busy with other trauma patients, he decided that Dr.Tran and I would do the surgery.

By the time the surgical team—nurses, technicians, cleaners and anesthesiologist—was ready, it was 5 am. Dr. Tran had been patiently sitting on a lounge chair with his eyes closed, waiting.

***

I'd seen a burr hole surgery done in medical school, and I had assisted in a few while on the neurosurgery service at VMC. One of them, which I remembered vividly, was with Dr. Slater, a neurosurgeon in town who helped out at VMC. He was one of the voluntary staff surgeons who worked without getting paid or any other form of compensation. They just did it because it was the right thing to do.

One night when I was on call, we had a patient with a subdural hematoma who needed surgery, so I contacted the neurosurgeon on call. It was Dr. Slater.

Dr. Slater arrived at 2 am, ready for surgery. He was an athletic man in his late 40s or early 50s with a crew cut, wearing a pair of dark-rimmed glasses. I always looked forward to working with him. He was happy as usual and full of funny things to tell me—the lowly intern.

As we were scrubbing, with a smile on his face and mischief in his eyes, he told me this joke that I would always remember—as well as Dr. Slater's grinning face—and laugh every time I thought of it.

This guy wakes up one morning to find a gorilla in his tree. He looks in the phone book for a gorilla removal service until he finds one.

"Is it a boy or girl gorilla?" the service guy asks.

"Boy," is the man's response.

"Oh yeah, I can do it. I'll be right there," says the service guy.

with hooks. The skin was pulled away from the surgery site and kept in place with special clips.

"James, as you know, the scalp is very vascular, so stopping the bleeding is important so you can see the skull clearly," Dr. Tran explained.

With the electro-cautery, I carefully stopped the bleeding. Dr. Tran then handed me the manual drill, saying, "I'm sure you'll know how to use this drill."

"I've assisted in several craniotomies and have used the drill before," I confirmed, taking it from him.

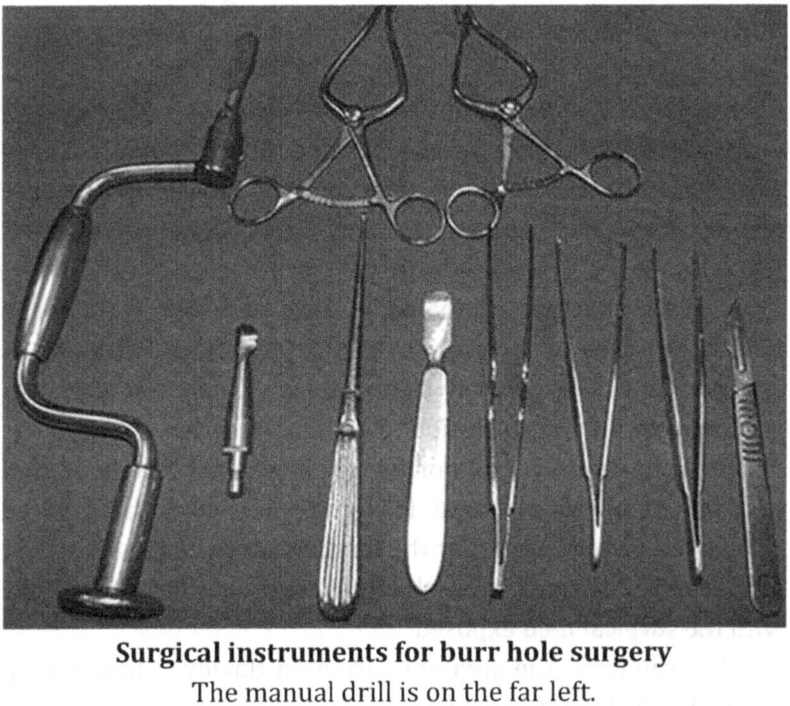

Surgical instruments for burr hole surgery
The manual drill is on the far left.

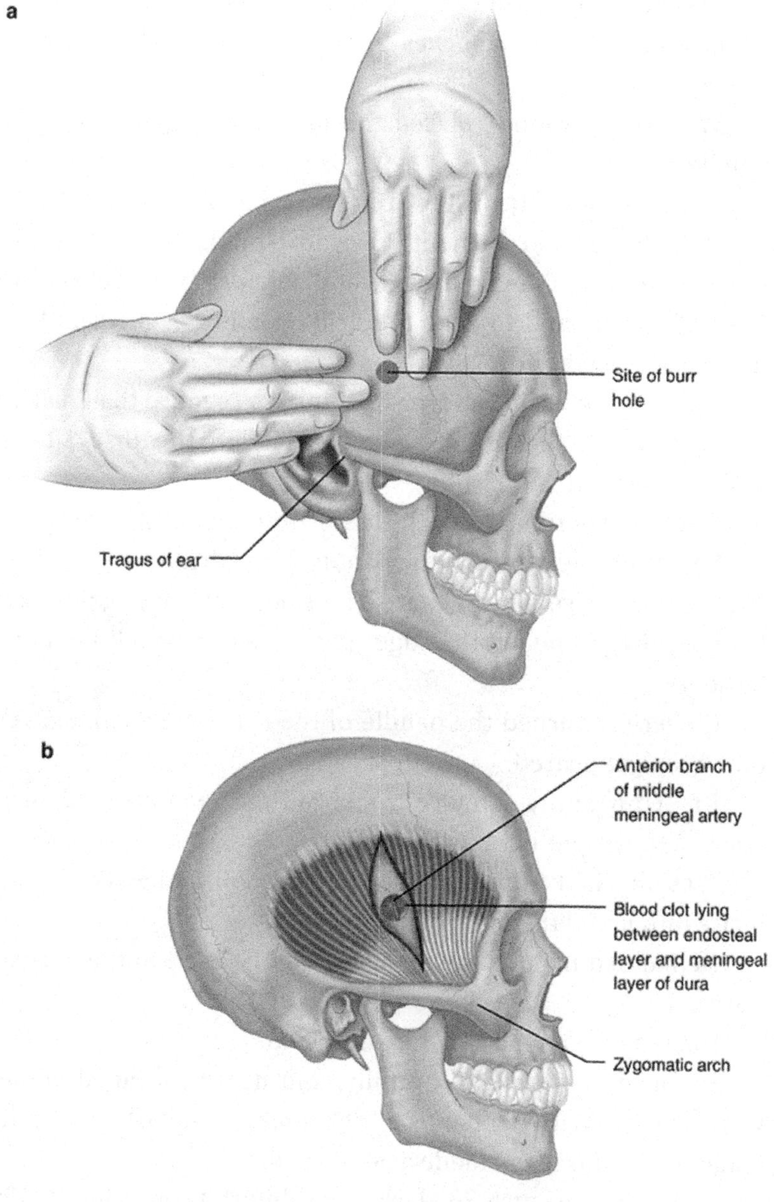

Burr Hole Surgery

"This is where you can start drilling," he said as he pointed to an area about two inches above and one inch anterior to Hayley's right ear.

With trepidation, I placed the drill and began turning the handle.

"You can be a little faster," Dr. Tran smiled.

With his encouragement, I began turning the handle with more speed. Dr. Tran squirted water to rinse bone debris from the drilling site and to keep the drill cool. But at the rate I was drilling, there was little heat.

"Let's check," said Dr. Tran. "I think we're more than halfway through." With the bright light focused on the drill site, he looked carefully.

"You can continue, and a little slower now," he advised.

So, I continued turning the handle of the drill.

"I think we're almost there," he said, checking again. Using his index finger, he felt the edges of the hole. "Just a little more," he added.

Gingerly, I turned the handle of the drill, and soon a silvery membrane appeared.

Dr. Tran sprayed more water on the wound, and again focused the bright light on the hole.

"Yes, this is the dura matter," he said. "All we need to do is to incise into it and the old blood will drain."

He handed me the scalpel again, and pointed to the exposed dura.

"Just make an incision," he instructed.

I looked at the dura carefully, and noted no blood vessels were around. With my hands a little shaky, I gingerly placed the blade on the dura, and made a gentle stab.

There was a gush of dark red, almost brown fluid. With cotton gauze, we dried the area. There was no more fluid leaking from the hole. We waited, and saw no signs of any new bleeding. Whatever had caused the bleeding had stopped.

The hole was covered with the scalp. I placed about ten thick black silk sutures to re-approximate the scalp incision that had been pulled away. The edges of the surgical wound looked even.

"You have done your first burr hole surgery. Congratulations," Dr. Tran exclaimed.

I smiled with satisfaction, thinking that if I were at a reservation hospital with a patient with subdural hematoma, I'd be able to save that person's life if there wasn't a neurosurgeon around.

After surgery, I made rounds of the patients on the ward. I stopped by the ICU just as Hayley was coming out of anesthesia.

As I was on call Friday, I got to go home after checking up on the patients on the floor.

I was anxious to see Hayley on Sunday. She was on the ward, sitting up in her bed watching TV, with her mother sitting next to her. She barely remembered me, as she'd been confused when I initially saw her.

"Hi Hayley," I said, re-introducing myself. "You may not remember me. I'm so glad you're responding to the surgery so well. The pressure in your brain has been released," I explained.

"Yes, my mom told me what happened and what you guys did. I'm feeling really good," she replied with a big smile.

I then did a neurological examination, checking her reflexes. Her pupils were round and reactive. I looked inside her eyes, and saw that the optic nerves were normal. I asked her questions to test her mental status such as the month and year, simple additions and subtractions, and who was the president, etc. She responded correctly, much to my relief and pride.

I will always remember Hayley and my first burr hole surgery.

Chapter 3
Code Blue

I WAS TWO WEEKS INTO MY INTERNAL MEDICINE ROTATION during my internship. Most of the interns had taken the ACLS—Advanced Cardiac Life Support—course in which we learned to treat patients who had cardiac arrests and failed to respond to initial shocks, and those whose hearts weren't fibrillating. The ACLS method involved intra-venous fluids, medications such as epinephrine and invasive procedures such a placing central IV lines. Generally it was much more difficult to start an IV on a patient who was in cardiac arrest because the blood had stopped flowing.

Donna May Reed Katarian was a well-known patient on the medicine floor. Even though she had private insurance and was well-to-do, she chose to come to the county hospital because she liked the attending physician, an endocrinologist who had been treating her diabetes for many years.

Donna May was not Armenian as her last name suggested. She was an Okie. Her parents had left Oklahoma during the Dust Bowl drought and headed west to find work because the situation at home was so desperate. They initially landed in the Monterey-Salinas area in coastal California (made famous by John Steinbeck) to work in the lettuce fields. Later the family moved to the foothills near the Fresno area in a small town called Porterville. Donna May married her high school sweetheart, a handsome Armenian whose family owned many acres of vineyard and a packinghouse.

I met Donna May on the first day of my internal medicine rotation during one of her admissions and was impressed by her humor, resiliency and her will to hang on to life. She was admitted for a reevaluation of her very labile blood sugar, which hit extreme highs and lows in a short time, causing her to pass out or feel very strange—as she put it, "I'm just not feeling myself." She talked about the several Jaguars she and her husband owned, and the numerous cruises they'd been on. She also often talked about her two daughters, aged twelve and fourteen. The younger daughter was born with hydrocephaly and her shunts frequently plugged up and required surgeries to reopen them or to put in new ones.

Life hadn't been easy for Donna. She'd lived with diabetes since she was eight, and after almost thirty years she was suffering from the many complications of the disease. She had developed peripheral neuropathy and would experience a "pins and needles" sensation in her feet whenever she walked, and sometimes even when she wasn't walking. Her eyes had developed retinopathy and she'd received laser treatments at Stanford University. Her kidneys had stopped working and she had scratch marks all over her arms and neck from the itching caused by renal failure. With help from her husband and sister, she'd been getting peritoneal dialysis at home, which involved infusing gallons of saline solution into her abdominal cavity daily to get rid of the waste her kidneys were no longer able to filter. In spite of all these problems, I'd never seen her sad, and she often remarked, "I am going to lick this."

She was a petite woman with coarse blond hair, light blue eyes and light brown eyebrows. As I got close to examine her retina I could smell her "acetone breath," the sweet-smelling breath of a diabetic when their sugar is too high. Her skin was dry to the touch and showed a certain shade that had been described as "frosted with ice." She always had her hair coiffured and her nails painted, and she usually wore a hint of a pleasant-smelling perfume—normally I disliked perfumes because of my allergy to them.

On this visit to the hospital Donna was very sick and was barely responsive when her husband brought her in. Her blood sugar was over six hundred, which I'd never seen in any patient—normally it should be around one hundred. She was admitted to the "large room" next to the nurses' station for close observation. The large room was for seriously ill patients before they were admitted to the ICU.

I was on call that night, and at ten o'clock I was already very much behind in my work. I'd gone down to the basement cafeteria for a quick cup of coffee and to go over my list of chores, getting organized and planning how to tackle them as efficiently as I could. The nightly news on the TV in one corner of the cafeteria was just coming on when a Code Blue was announced over the PA.

I ran up the stairs to the third floor and into the large room.

I'd never been directly involved with a Code Blue before. I had observed a few as a medical student at the Douglas County Hospital in Omaha during my internal medicine rotation. With so many medical students, interns, residents and nurses, I could barely see the patient during the chaos. But I had watched a teaching video of a simulated code a few times, and had gone over in my mind how I would conduct one if it happened. I had practiced doing the compressions on a mannequin.

During my rotation in the ER, many CPRs were performed. The ER residents would usually lead the resuscitative effort. The interns were usually busy with other patients who didn't have life-threatening problems. When we weren't busy, we would participate in the activity, mostly as assistants and not directly involved in the resuscitative effort.

Dan Sinisky, my favorite senior resident, was already in the room compressing Donna's chest. An easy-going Polish American from Chicago, Dan never seemed to get excited or angry with anybody. About my height, he had a thick mop of sandy hair that fell to his shoulders and across his forehead to just above his eyebrows. He often flashed a toothy smile that made his broad, square face seem even broader. It was reassuring to see him there. As the most senior physician present and a member of Donna's treatment team, he naturally became the code leader.

Unlike a university teaching hospital, VMC rarely had medical students, which I was grateful for. Just out of medical school myself, I was trying to learn as much as I could and didn't think I knew enough yet to teach others. I was already far too busy and didn't need another demand on my precious time. I felt relieved that it was just me, Dan and a few nurses and technicians, and not chaotic like some of the Code Blues I'd observed in Omaha, with numerous medical students running around and different people shouting orders. I had found all the confusion nerve wracking.

Karen, the head nurse, had already pushed the red crash cart into the room. Donna was already hooked up to the cardiac monitor, which had sounded an alarm when her heart went into ventricular fibrillation (V-fib). Now the machine showed us that her heart was contracting in an uncoordinated manner, quivering rather than pumping blood.

Karen had obviously done this a few times before and was deftly cutting the plastic locks that secured the drawers and the defibrillator paddles. I helped Karen roll Donna onto a wooden board. As soon as the board was under her, I began compressing with a firm and deliberate pressure, making sure that I wasn't directly over her sternum as had been stressed in the teaching video. Another nurse cranked the bed adjustment lever in a counterclockwise direction and tilted Donna's head down in the

"Trendelenburg" position to encourage blood from the feet and legs to flow toward the brain. I counted "one thousand one, one thousand two... " and after five compressions, paused. Dan was now at the head of the bed with the resuscitation bag, giving Donna two puffs of air when I paused. As I continued the compressions, Dan narrowed his eyelids, straining as he looked at the cardiac monitor screen. Soon the respiratory therapist arrived and took over on the resuscitation bag.

The monitor continued to show limp squiggles and not the higher waves we were hoping for. By this time Dan had the paddles—now charged—in his hands and he yelled, "200 joules and everyone stand back!" He pressed a large red button and a jolt was delivered. Donna shuddered, but there was no change on the monitor.

"Epi!" Dan yelled. Karen swiftly withdrew from a vial of epinephrine and injected it into the IV line that had been put in earlier that morning.

"Lidocaine!" Dan shouted. Karen withdrew from a vial of Lidocaine and injected it into the IV line.

As I continued compressions on Donna's chest, every push was causing her torso to shift on the board under her. The gravity of the Trendelenburg position was also causing her to drift toward the head of the bed. I dragged her body and tried to center her on the board.

Dan probably noticed that my arms were getting tired and suggested that he take over the compressions.

"Jim, how about blood gas?" Dan cried. Karen handed me a glass syringe with a long needle. I tried to palpate the femoral artery and made a stab and withdrew. The blood was so dark that it was obvious it wasn't getting oxygenated.

Blood gas is to evaluate how oxygenated the arterial blood is. It is done by using a long needle to get to an artery, usually the femoral, but sometimes the radial artery.

I resumed compressions, and Dan reapplied the paddles to Donna's chest and delivered another jolt, this time 300 joules. With more power from the defibrillator, Donna shook more this time. But nothing happened on the monitor.

"More Epi!" Dan barked again. Karen withdrew from another vial and injected it into the IV.

Dan delivered another jolt, and this time it was 350 joules. Nothing happened on the monitor, still just the low squiggly lines.

"Bicarb!" Dan shouted. This was almost the cookbook sequence we'd learned to follow in an attempt to restart the heart. By now the unoxygenated blood had become acidic. The rationale for adding bicarbonate was to make it less acidic and slow down the damage to the cells. Karen injected the bicarbonate. But nothing seemed to work and the monitor continued to show the same low squiggly line.

Now a young nurse who had just come on for her 11 pm shift joined in and took over the chest compressions.

By now we'd been working on Donna for more than half an hour, and my arms were really tired.

"Jim, what do you think? " Dan asked me.

I was a little surprised by his question. I was just the intern and he had a great deal more experience than I did—perhaps it was a show of respect. I'd read about calcium and thought we had nothing to lose, so in a tired voice I said, "How about calcium?"

"Calcium!" Dan yelled. Karen withdrew from a vial and injected the solution into the IV. It was becoming obvious that we had worked on Donna long enough and we weren't going to bring a dead person back to life.

Dan gave Donna another jolt and yelled, "More Epi!" The waves on the monitor were looking more like a flat line now, indicating no activity in the heart.

"Atropine," said Dan in a dispirited voice, now tired and grasping at straws. He was giving Donna everything in the book. Karen dutifully withdrew from a vial of Atropine and injected it into the IV. Nothing happened.

Dan gave Donna another jolt. The monitor continued to show essentially a flat line. From the shape of the wave on the monitor, even with my limited knowledge of cardiology, I suspected there wasn't even a glimmer of hope that her heart might restart.

After about forty-five minutes Dan declared, "I think we've done enough." Karen agreed and put the vial of Atropine she had in her hand back into the drawer of the red crash cart. I too nodded my head in agreement.

By now the room was a mess with tracings of the cardiac monitor strewn all over. The needles, empty vials and syringes were collected and put into a plastic container. It would be the intern's job to document what had been done and that would take another hour. At least it wasn't my job to call the family.

During recent years ACLS has become controversial. Statistics for such heroic attempts were dismal. They were rarely successful. The thinking now is that the heart stops because the organs can no longer continue. The few successes were usually healthy individuals whose hearts had suddenly stopped because of arrhythmia and not those individuals whose hearts stopped because of end-stage chronic disease. But ACLS had become a norm because there were no other options. If there was a cardiac arrest and nothing was done, the plaintiff's attorney would have a field day. No physician would risk not doing the resuscitation even though the success rate was so very low.

Perhaps my medical training had succeeded in shaping me into a professional with a sense of detached concern—strangely, I wasn't devastated by our failure to revive Donna. Even during the code I felt that I was doing my job and had prepared myself well for it by rehearsing, viewing videos of the procedure, going through the steps mentally and knowing by heart the various medications and their indications. I felt that I had worked hard trying to revive her. Oddly, I didn't grieve Donna's passing. I asked myself what there was to salvage in a person with such advanced diabetes and so many complications. What kind of life would she have had if we succeeded in reviving her? Her heart had stopped for a reason. Even if we were able to restart the heart this time, it would most likely stop again for the same reason.

Perhaps I was just trying not to let the incident bother me. I came up with all kinds of reasons why Donna might not have wanted to be revived. Perhaps perversely, I became aware that I actually enjoyed doing the code, in the respect that I'd been able to perform under pressure and I felt that this was what being a physician was all about. Of course I felt bad that Donna had died so young. I reminded myself that life was unfair, and in spite of all the medical knowledge in the world, it was indeed still a mystery.

I couldn't understand why I was having such peculiar thoughts and feeling a little detached. It dawned on me that people worked so hard to become doctors because they could do something that others couldn't. I'd heard that doctors earned their power through suffering. Perhaps through the suffering of hard work and humiliation during our almost punitive training, we felt that we'd paid our dues and should be special.

In spite of being exhausted and behind in my work, I felt a vague sense of vindication that I had persisted in my goal to become a physician even when things didn't look good. I thought about the books I liked to read about physicians, which I was attracted to because of the nebulous feeling of romance surrounding the idea of being a doctor. Strangely, I seemed to be experiencing a quiet satisfaction in my misery—having to work so hard with no prospect of any sleep for the night, but glad that I was becoming a physician. It was now 3 am and I was still trying to complete my long list of chores.

There was little chance that I'd get any sleep at all before I began another day of work, but I carried on, feeling satisfied that we'd done the very best we could for Donna.

Chapter 4
The Burn Patient

IT WAS LATE ONE FRIDAY AFTERNOON and the other interns were signing out their patients to me. They were getting ready to enjoy a free weekend, or at least a free Friday night. I was on call and trying to get psyched up for another busy Friday night, which usually included caring for stabbing and shooting victims from many of the clubs in west Fresno. But I wasn't prepared for what turned out to be the most traumatic event of my entire internship.

During dinner the Burn Center nurse called to let me know that the helicopter was bringing in a patient with extensive third degree burns from a Bakersfield area refinery. There had been an explosion and the unfortunate welder was immediately engulfed in flames, which were shortly put out by his coworkers. From my limited experience with burn patients, I knew that those with such severe and extensive burns usually didn't do well.

The Burn Center at VMC was the first in Central California and had opened with great fanfare just a year earlier. The new director, a good-looking young surgeon with dark hair and a strong resemblance to Dr. Kildare (Richard Chamberlain), had just finished his fellowship in plastic surgery at the Vancouver General Hospital affiliated with the University of British Columbia Medical School. From the onset, he complained to the residents and interns that this was not what he had in mind. He was interested in reconstructive surgery and not a burn unit and felt that the head of the hospital had misrepresented the nature of the job.

There were already two burn patients in the Center who were recovering slowly but steadily from non-life-threatening burns. I could tell that the director, Dr. Harrison, would rather be doing surgery than treating the burn patients, which required a great deal of knowledge in physiology and the science of fluid replacement. What usually kills a severely burned victim is the loss of bodily fluids leading to shock. When a great deal of fluid has been lost in a short time, the body experiences a sudden shift of electrolytes. This leads to great instability in many organs, including the heart—which can sometimes lead to arrhythmias.

Soon the patient, Mr. Bergdahl, a stocky man in his mid-forties, arrived. Severe swelling had set in, obscuring his facial features and making him look bloated. He'd been given morphine for the pain and didn't seem to be in any discomfort. Under swollen lids I could see fear in his light blue eyes.

Randy, the muscular young head nurse, with the help of an aide, carefully moved Mr. Bergdahl from the gurney to the bed. The three of us began the slow process of cleaning up the skin, removing the dead skin, leaving the blisters alone, then placing a thin, gauze-like material with petrolatum over the exposed surface of the deeper layer of skin. Mr. Bergdahl had an oxygen mask on, which he tried to adjust occasionally.

Dr. Harrison stopped by and talked to us, examined the patient, made some notes on the chart and wrote some orders, including one for a central venous line. He looked at the cardiac monitor and then went home.

A central venous catheter, also known as a central line, is a tube that is placed in a large vein in the neck, chest, groin, or arm to give fluids, blood or medications, or to do medical tests quickly.

Randy brought out a minor surgery tray and handed me the necessary instruments. With trepidation, I carefully palpated Mr. Bergdahl's right clavicle area. This was a blind procedure, meaning I couldn't actually see the subclavian vein and would insert the catheter without actually knowing if I were in the correction position. This procedure carried risks such as pneumothorax, i.e, collapsing the lung, which would be disastrous.

I'd done two such procedures with supervision before. With the rest of the surgical residents busy taking care of trauma patients, none of them were available to come to the Burn Center. As Mr. Bergdahl's condition was critical and he needed fluids quickly, I decided to go ahead with the procedure.

Saying a few prayers, I pushed the catheter through the skin and advanced it a little further. To my relief, blood dripped from the catheter and I knew I was in the right place.

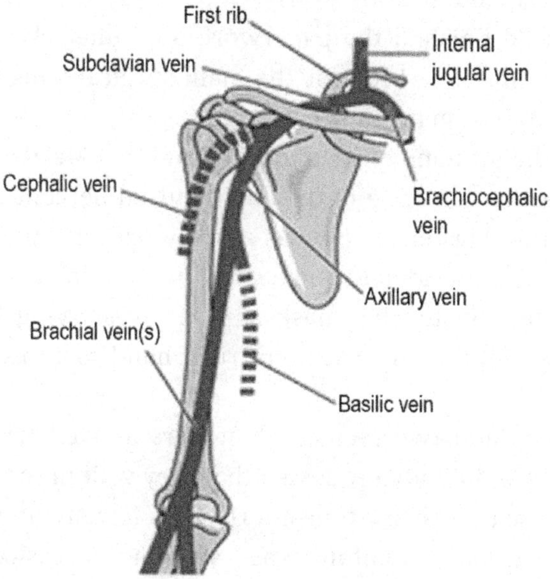

Anatomy of the Subclavian Vein

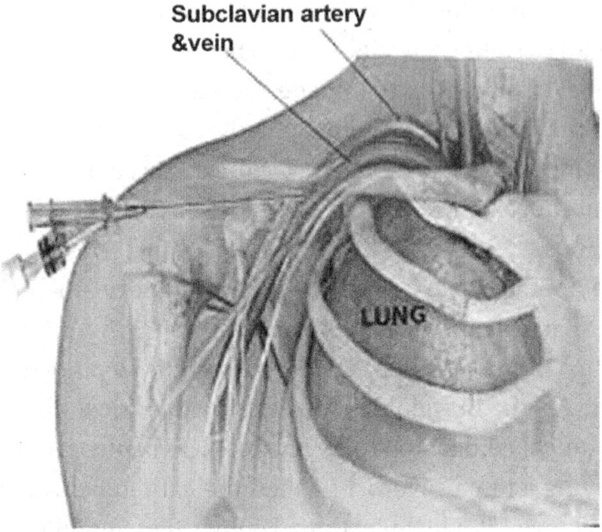

Placement of a central venous catheter

Randy got out a bag of plasma and hung it on the IV pole, and it began to drip into the line slowly.

When I'd finished the paperwork and other chores for the patient's admission, I left for the main surgical wing to tend to the other duties on my long list.

At midnight Randy paged me and said that Mr. Bergdahl was getting restless. In spite of the one hundred percent oxygen, he was breathing faster. As he was already on a morphine drip to help the pain, I decided to add a small dose of Valium to ease his anxiety. He adjusted his mask as if he was trying to tell me something. But then he waved his right hand as if to say, "Never mind."

His wife and two teenage daughters arrived. They visited him briefly and Randy requested that they wait in the lobby and visit him one person at a time hourly, for a few minutes only.

The cardiac monitor was showing occasional PVCs (Premature Ventricular Contractions) and his heart rate had increased to over ninety beats per minute. I tried to call the two residents who were also covering the Center, but they were in surgery with a traffic accident victim who had a fractured pelvis and internal bleeding.

An hour went by and the frequency of Mr. Bergdahl's PVCs had increased to four or five per minute, and he was again trying to tell me something, pointing his finger to the oxygen mask. But then he stopped, closed his eyes and rested his head on the pillow.

At this point I felt very uncomfortable, realizing that this was beyond my expertise. I called Dr. Harrison. He instructed me to increase the infusion rate of the plasma and to start another 250cc bag in two hours. In the meantime, I was trying to read about the complicated formula for replacing lost fluids in burn patients. It warned of inadequate as well as too much fluid in the body. As I was talking with Dr. Harrison I detected some indecisiveness, as if he too was uncomfortable with the situation. He had just finished his fellowship in plastic surgery and I didn't know how much experience he had with severely burned patients.

I again tried to call the residents, but they were still in surgery. As Dr. Harrison was the attending physician and above the residents in authority, I had to be careful that I was following the chain of command in my request for help. More PVCs showed up on the monitor. I again called Dr. Harrison and he ordered a Lidocaine drip in an attempt to stabilize the heart and perhaps stop the PVCs.

It was now 2 am and I was feeling really uneasy. I sat in a chair next to the bed and watched Mr. Bergdahl, trying to comprehend the situation, unable to shake off a feeling of foreboding.

I was still there at 3 am, nervously watching the cardiac monitor. Mr. Bergdahl's heart rate had now gone up to a hundred and the PVCs had increased to over six per minute. I couldn't shake the feeling that something bad was going to happen to Mr. Bergdahl, but I didn't know what do to. Feeling like a pest, I again called Dr. Harrison and told him that I was really worried.

"I'll come in right away," he said before I could even finish my sentence. I felt a great sense of relief.

As Dr. Harrison was putting on a gown and mask to enter the room, the cardiac monitor alarm went off and we saw that the heartbeat pattern had become a squiggly line—indicating ventricular fibrillation—and Mr. Bergdahl went limp. Then the monitor showed a flat line (asystole)—his heart had stopped beating.

Randy called a Code Blue, and immediately began chest compressions. Dr. Harrison got the resuscitation bag and began forcing air into Mr. Bergdahl's lungs. Soon the respiratory therapist arrived and took over. Dr. Harrison asked me to page an anesthesiologist—I thought perhaps he was planning to intubate Mr. Bergdahl.

To me, the activity at this point seemed futile. What could we do now that we couldn't do when Mr. Bergdahl was still alive? We gave Mr. Bergdahl almost every drug in the red crash cart. The monitor continued to show a flat line. Forty-five minutes later we quit working on him.

While all this was happening, Mrs. Bergdahl and her two girls were at the opposite side of the building in the lobby, unaware of what was going on. I couldn't imagine having to talk to them. Dr. Harrison told me he would go talk to the family.

By the time I finished with the paperwork it was 5 am. I went outside to the garden between the two wings of the hospital. The moon, still in the sky, was bright and round. It was a cold morning and I sat down on a bench, put my head in my hands and rested it on the picnic table in front of me. I was more confused than anything. I shook my head, as if it were possible to forget the vision of Mr. Bergdahl as I'd watched him from the chair next to his bed. I tried to tell myself that this wasn't real, it had just been a bad dream. It was as if I'd watched a train wreck in slow motion and there wasn't a thing I could do. Perhaps nothing would have helped, not the best burn specialist, not the best cardiologist, not the best physiologist or pharmacologist who knew just the right solutions and drugs to give Mr. Bergdahl. Perhaps in this case his body had been so badly damaged that it was beyond repair, and there was simply nothing we could've done to save this man's life.

I had been at his side almost the entire time, sadly and helplessly watching him die in front of my eyes.

Soon it was 6 am and breakfast was being served in the cafeteria. I got a tray and took my food back outside. I must have been hungry, but I couldn't eat and instead drank the black coffee. I just wanted some solitude.

It was now 7 am Saturday morning. Nina, the intern on call for the day, found me still sitting in the cold.

"I heard about the burn patient," she said with a sympathetic look.

"It was a rough night," I replied in a barely audible voice, emotionally drained. She was briefed on my other patients and I signed out to her.

Even though Mr. Bergdahl's death occurred almost fifty years ago, I can still vividly see the fright in his eyes and often wonder what he'd been trying to tell me that tragic day.

Chapter 5
Peter

PART OF MY INTERNSHIP was a two-week rotation on the gastroenterology service. By now, I was tired of internal medicine and all the patients with chronic medical problems. Many of the patients on this service had irritable colon, and the rest were men with cirrhosis of the liver from alcoholism.

Even during my short stint on this service, I'd seen several patients who had been in and out of the hospital for the same reasons. It was like a revolving door. They were in the hospital for a week or so, got cleaned up and discharged, only to return with the same problem a few weeks later. It was frustrating because such patients took up so much time, and sadly, it didn't seem like we helped them that much.

Having grown up in a culture where people rarely drank, and almost nobody drank in excess to the point of getting cirrhosis, it puzzled me how so many men were drinking themselves to death.

I learned that cirrhosis is a late stage of scarring (fibrosis) of the liver caused by many forms of liver diseases and conditions, such as hepatitis and chronic alcoholism.

Each time the liver is injured—whether by disease, excessive alcohol consumption or another cause—it tries to repair itself. In the process, scar tissue forms. As cirrhosis progresses, more and more scar tissue forms, making it difficult for the liver to function (decompensated cirrhosis). Advanced cirrhosis is life-threatening.

The liver damage done by cirrhosis generally can't be undone. But if it's diagnosed early and the cause is treated, further damage can be limited and, in rare instances, reversed.

In people who have cirrhosis, high blood pressure in the veins that carry blood from the intestines to the liver (portal hypertension) causes many problems. One serious complication of portal hypertension is variceal bleeding.

When blood pressure increases in the portal vein system, veins in the esophagus, stomach and rectum enlarge to accommodate blocked blood flow through the liver. The presence of enlarged veins (varices) usually causes no symptoms early on.

As the blood pressure in the portal vein system continues to increase, the walls of these expanded veins become thinner, causing the veins to rupture and bleed. This is called variceal bleeding. The more severe the liver damage and the larger the varices, the greater the risk is for variceal bleeding. If varices aren't treated, bleeding can lead to death.

Treatment for variceal bleeding can be challenging and may include medicines as well as endoscopic therapy (endoscopic banding or sclerotherapy).

A failing liver can't make enough clotting factors, which help blood to clot. Bleeding in the gastrointestinal tract is common with this condition.

Cirrhosis often has no signs or symptoms until liver damage is extensive. When signs and symptoms do occur, they may include fatigue and bleeding or bruising easily.

Peter, in his mid-thirties, was a chubby man with a huge round face that looked bloated and puffy. He had all the signs of an alcoholic. His nose was large, red and bumpy with prominent blood vessels, which are known as telangiectasia.

One of the earliest signs of alcohol abuse is a persistently red face due to enlarged blood vessels (telangiectasia). This appears because regulation of vascular control in the brain fails with sustained alcohol intake.

The head of gastroenterology, Dr. Peter Roberts, was a tall handsome man with a resemblance to the famous preacher Billy Graham. He was an excellent teacher and usually full of confidence. He could pass a tube into the stomach of any patient in seconds. When Peter's massive bleeding began, I could see fear in Dr. Roberts' eyes as he poured more and more ice-cold water into Peter's stomach tube, trying to stop the bleeding.

The bleeding continued and Dr. Roberts inserted a tube with balloons inflated at the end to apply pressure to the engorged veins in Peter's esophagus. But still the bleeding continued. Dr. Roberts seemed to be running out of options to help Peter. As a lowly intern I could only watch as the specialist and residents tried to save this poor man's life.

Next, a central IV line was successfully put into his chest by a surgical resident and units of blood were poured into Peter. After what seemed like an eternity, the bleeding finally stopped.

After another week at the hospital Peter was discharged and sent home. While he was in the hospital, a psychologist and a social worker both worked with him to try to stop his drinking.

He was referred to the surgical service for evaluation to have a porta-caval shunt procedure. This procedure involved connecting the portal vein to the inferior vena cava, which takes blood from the organs and lower limbs to the heart. By making this new connection, blood would bypass the liver and reduce the blood pressure in the liver.

It just happened that I was getting off the Gastroenterology service and on to my four months of general surgery rotation when Peter and I again crossed paths.

His case was brought up in grand round, and the pros and cons of this surgery for Peter were discussed at great length. Some felt that because of Peter's long history of alcoholism, it was unlikely that he would stop drinking, which would make the surgery pointless.

The new chief of surgery happened to specialize in such surgeries and felt that Peter should be given a chance so he wouldn't bleed anymore and could lead a more normal life, and even return to work.

After lengthy discussions, the majority felt Peter would benefit from the surgery. At that point, I wondered if, because it was a training program, the chief resident wanted more surgical experience and voted for the procedure.

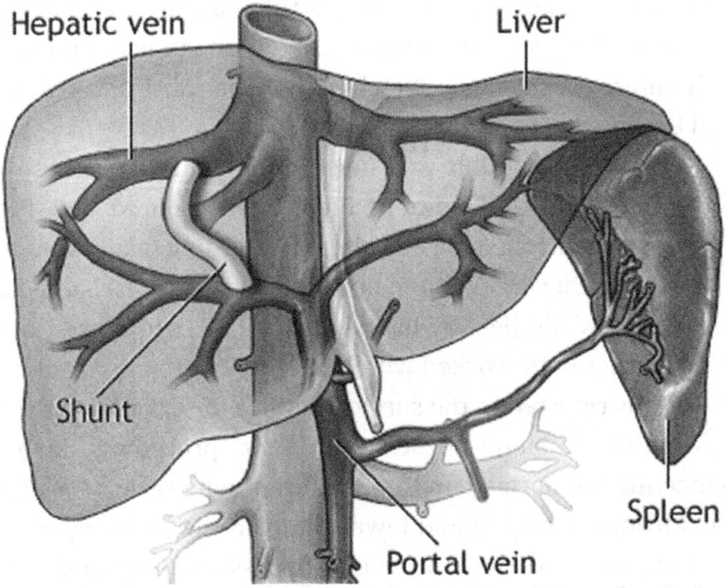

The shunt connecting the Hepatic vein to Portal vein is made of synthetic material such as Dacron

I was one of the five people who scrubbed in for the surgery. It was a very difficult procedure because it was so challenging to expose the various veins, and they were so friable. I tried to get a view of the veins, but I simply couldn't see them.

The surgery was complicated by excessive bleeding because Peter's failing liver couldn't make enough clotting factors, which help the blood to clot.

The chief of surgery, whose name interestingly was Dr. Robert Peters, just the reverse sequence of the gastroenterologist, worked really hard. It was fascinating to watch how he could connect a synthetic tube to two veins without a leak. But he did it.

After six long hours, the surgery was finished, and Dr. Peters declared it a success.

Peter was transferred to the ICU, where he remained for five days. Each day he was visited by a team of surgeons as well as the social worker and psychologist, counseling him not to drink anymore. After another five days on the ward, he was sent home.

Two months later, I was examining a patient in the ER with a hand injury involving a cut tendon, when the ambulance brought in a patient who had been vomiting copious amount of blood and was found unresponsive at his home in Tranquility, a small town in the valley.

The ambulance attendants performed CPR but they couldn't revive him.

The man was Peter. He had had a massive hemorrhage during another drinking binge and he simply bled to death.

He was thirty-five.

I couldn't get over the fact that this man knew he was drinking himself to death but he would not or could not stop.

Chapter 6
A Sliced Thumb

DURING THE SECOND HALF of my very stressful internship, in January of 1975, I began suffering severe abdominal pain. It lasted for weeks, but I continued working for fear of being labeled a slacker among the intern group, as my not working would add to their already heavy workload. When I began passing out because of the excruciating pain, I sought help. X-rays showed severe swelling of my intestines and bowel obstruction, and surgery was needed to rule out cancer. This was before the days of endoscopy.

I had major abdominal surgery and multiple biopsies were taken from my intestines. The diagnosis was a rare illness called Eosinophilic Gastro-enteritis, an autoimmune condition that was thought to be stress-related. Interestingly, similar cases had also been reported in other medical interns.

Before my illness, my plan was to return to the University of Nebraska for my orthopedic residency after my internship.

During this time there was a crisis in medical malpractice in California; some orthopedic and neurosurgeons were paying a few hundred thousand dollars a year for their coverage. It made headlines in the paper day after day. With my illness and the malpractice crisis, I was beginning to think that orthopedics might not be a good specialty to go into.

While recuperating from my surgery, I came across an advertisement for a new Family Practice Residency Program with affiliation to a major medical school, in Salinas, California.

The program had just been formed and they were looking for a few second-year house staff—the hospital had never had an internship program before. The program, including the internship, would be three years. After talking to the program head and visiting the facility, I was offered—and accepted—the position as chief resident. There would be six interns working under me.

Mary and I loved the California Central Coast area. Next to the hospital was a group of single story apartments, and the head of the residency program told us that we would get the three-bedroom end unit apartment with a washer and dryer in it, probably as an added incentive! I reasoned that if I still wanted to be a specialist I could move on after my residency. Another year of general medicine would help me gain more experience.

We read up on the Salinas area and learned that it was named for a nearby salt marsh and that it was the lettuce capital of the world. I also learned the names of the different kinds of lettuce grown in the area such as iceberg, Romaine, butter-head, loose-leaf types and so on.

I was surprised to learn that at one time, Monterey was the capital of California and had been under military rule after the signing of the Treaty of Guadalupe-Hidalgo at the end of the Mexican-American war.

In 1924, Salinas had the highest per capita income of any city in the United States.

Salinas is also the hometown of writer and Nobel Prize laureate John Steinbeck. The movie *East of Eden*, based on one of Steinbeck's books, was set in Salinas and the story was tangentially about the lettuce business in the area.

The name of the County Hospital was Natividad Medical Center. It was a smaller version of VMC, serving basically the same kinds of patients: all those who could not or would not go to the private sector. Much like Fresno, most of the agricultural workers were Mexicans, but this area also had a sizable population of Filipinos.

Our new apartment was the most desirable unit in the building, and with the washer and dryer was the greatest luxury we'd ever had. Our daughter Melissa, now two, had her own room and I used the extra room for my study. Behind the building was a small patch of land on which I grew several rows of turnips and radishes. The other five apartments were occupied by the interns.

The Family Practice Program was brand new and had been established in response to the shortage of primary care physicians in California. The head of the program was a Cambridge-trained British pediatrician. Dr. Lex Hayward, aka Sexy Lexy, was a loquacious, handsome man with prematurely white hair, and one of the longest-winded people I knew. I felt that he was a genuinely good person who tried to please everyone but in the end pleased no one. Often when a decision needed to be made, a half hour of discussion—essentially a monologue posing the pros and cons—would drone on, eventually reaching a conclusion that could've been accomplished in less than five minutes.

I was given the official title of Chief Resident, since I was the only second-year person and also the only house staff with a medical license. None of the six interns could write prescriptions without a signature from me or one of the teaching faculty staff. To add to the confusion, not all the staff members were also teaching faculty. The surgery, ob/gyn and pediatrics departments each had one board-certified specialist, but I wasn't certain about the credentials of the staff in general medicine. Other specialists in departments like orthopedics, neurosurgery, urology, oral surgery, otolaryngology and ophthalmology were private physicians who had to be called in when needed.

Three times a week a noon-time conference was held, and I was responsible for making the arrangements and deciding on the topics.

About two months into the program I realized I'd made a mistake. I was the workhorse and a source of cheap labor for the hospital, but I wasn't learning from anyone. Each morning, to psych myself up to face the general clinic, I had to drink two large cups of strong coffee and listen to marching music by John Philip Sousa before I could take the five-minute walk to meet the throngs of waiting patients. The red lights above all eight rooms would be on, indicating that a patient was waiting in each room. Once at the clinic, I worked nonstop, going from one patient to another, not even sitting down.

In addition to the general clinic, I also had to take care of whatever came in through the ER. I prided myself that I could suture up a child's cut in five minutes and still do an excellent job.

By noon my head would be pounding and spinning and I would escape to hide in the nearby bushes where a small creek flowed to calm my nerves. By then I was drained and needed to recharge. In four hours I would have seen over 30 patients, and I needed some silence.

It was exceedingly stressful trying to manage so many patients with chronic diseases, many of whom had been patients at the clinic for years and never had a definitive management plan. How could anyone formulate a meaningful management plan when he had to see so many patients in an hour? There were many patients with chronic headaches who never had the proper workups. Each time, a patient's visit was much like the previous visit, usually ending with a prescription for more codeine pills. I lived in fear that some of them had more severe problems, but I didn't have the time to do the proper diagnostic workups. When I saw a patient with a headache, my own head began to ache from worrying that I might be sitting on a time bomb such as a brain tumor growing in the patient's head.

Many elderly people came in suffering from insomnia. When I didn't give them any medicine for sleep, their families often got angry. Grandma was keeping everybody up at night. When I did prescribe medicine for sleep, other members of the patients' families accused me of trying to turn Grandma into a drug addict. It was an impossible and often thankless job.

I was trying to manage the blood sugar levels of a diabetic woman, but she wouldn't follow the instructions for her diet and would not lose weight. She told me that she'd been drinking diet Pepsi and was surprised that she still hadn't lost any weight—she thought the diet Pepsi itself had ingredients that would actually cause weight loss!

During one visit, after her examination was finished, she stood up on the ledge of the examination table. As I was writing notes on her chart the table began tipping over beneath her weight, and she fell into my lap before I could stand up to help her, her right hand hitting my face and knocking my glasses to the floor. There was a loud crashing noise and everyone in the clinic rushed to see what had happened. She was embarrassed, but fortunately only her ego was hurt.

The patients with emphysema who continued to smoke were the most frustrating. A few times I almost lost my temper. How could I pretend to be taking care of these patients when I couldn't even make them value their own health? It was demoralizing.

I was truly disillusioned with primary care.

One Tuesday morning at about 11 am, a Mexican worker showed up at the ER after slicing off the tip of his left thumb while working in the lettuce fields. He was trying to keep pace with the machine that collected heads of lettuce into boxes. He was in a hurry and his very sharp knife got a little too close to his hand that was holding a head of lettuce, and he accidently sliced off the tip of his left thumb.

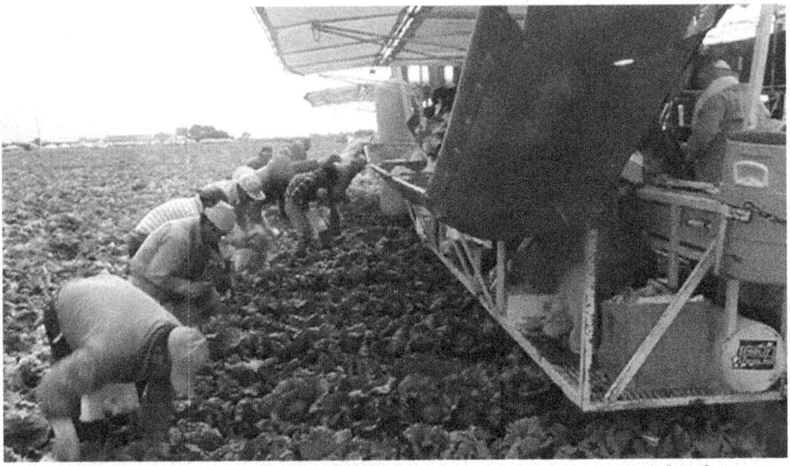

The harvesting rig (harvesting machine) is attached to a tractor that pulls the rig forward, and the harvesting crew needs to select the heads of lettuce that are of proper quality and harvest them at the same speed the harvesting rig is moving.

The best way to harvest lettuce is by using a sharp knife to cut the heads off the stalk when they're still firm.

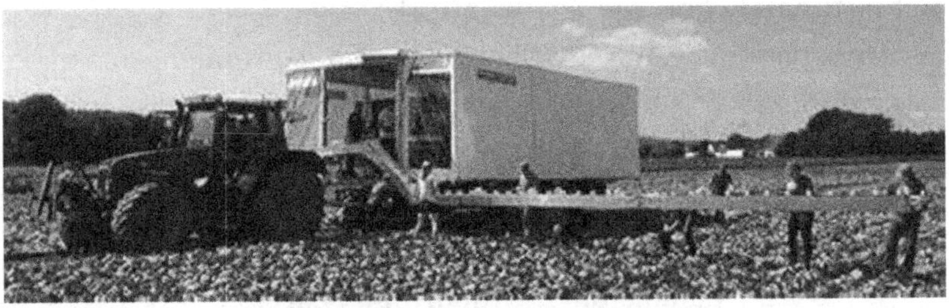

Harvesting Lettuce in Salinas

It wasn't a deep cut, just the skin and a thin layer of flesh. The bleeding had been stopped with a handkerchief tied at the base of the patient's thumb and he had another handkerchief wrapped around the thumb.

Javier was in his mid-twenties, a good looking man with a mustache, reminding me of Omar Sharif in the movie Dr. Zhivago. He looked scared.

"Tienes algún dolor?" I asked.

"Un poco," he replied.

As I was the chief resident, and the only general surgeon was grief-stricken after his wife passed away from ovarian cancer, he was letting me do all sorts of surgery, including breast biopsies and revision of keloid scar tissues.

I told Javier to lie down on the examination table. With his hand on a tray table, I examined his thumb carefully.

His foreman handed me a wet towel containing the sliced-off skin. It was jagged and seemed full of dirt. I decided that it wasn't possible to reattach the contaminated skin.

During the four months on the surgical service in my internship, I'd seen quite a few skin grafts in the burn unit. I was even allowed to do one under supervision once.

As usual, Chief of Surgery Dr. Olson was smoking his pipe in the doctor's lounge, paralyzed by the death of his wife. I presented the case to him, and he took a deep puff of smoke into his mouth, held it for a few seconds, and then exhaled it, saying, "Jim, you can go ahead and put a skin graft on the defect."

"Where do you think I should get the skin?" I asked.

"The forearm would be the best," he replied.

I nodded and returned to the ER. The foreman was still there, attentive and concerned. My Spanish had gone as far as it could and it was beyond my ability to explain what needed to be done. So I turned to the foreman for translation help.

I explained that the wound needed to be covered with a skin graft, otherwise it wouldn't heal properly, and Javier wouldn't be able to return to work if it didn't heal. The treatment was to take a small piece of skin from his forearm and graft it to cover the wound.

Javier nodded as the foreman relayed my explanation and he signed the consent for the procedure.

After anesthetizing an area on the forearm with Lidocaine, I scrubbed it with Betadine. I carefully dissected a quarter-sized piece of skin and put it in a saline solution. The thumb was anesthetized and washed thoroughly with saline solution.

I carefully placed the piece of skin over Javier's injured thumb and stitched the edges with fine sutures.

A few layers of gauze were placed over the site, followed by fluffy cotton balls, and the thumb was then wrapped. Javier's hand was placed in a sling to keep it elevated and prevent swelling, and I prescribed antibiotics to prevent an infection.

Ideally, a procedure like that should've been done by a general surgeon, a hand surgeon or a plastic surgeon, but this was a small county hospital, and sometimes the patient didn't have the luxury of choosing from the best physicians. I felt comfortable with the procedure and was satisfied that I did a good job.

Javier returned the following day for a follow-up. There was no sign of infection and the donor skin looked pink and healthy. I cleaned the edges of the wound with hydrogen peroxide. Cotton balls were again placed over the site, and the thumb was re-wrapped and his hand placed back in a sling.

Javier returned a few days later. The wound continued to heal and the donor skin continued to look good and viable.

Two weeks after the skin graft, the donor skin seemed fully attached to the thumb and well healed. I carefully removed most of the sutures, and left a few to be removed later, as I was feeling a little unsure if the donor skin was fully healed.

Javier returned in another two weeks, and I removed the rest of the sutures. He moved his thumb and rubbed his thumb with his index finger.

"Yes, I can feel it," he exclaimed with a big smile. He could move his thumb with ease.

The graft took and healed beautifully: a success!

It was a moment of revelation for me, to realize how much I liked doing surgery and how much I loathed seeing patients with chronic problems that I could do so little about. Being an impatient person, I like to see results fast, and surgery provided such results. I'm certainly not putting down primary care, because I know what an important job it is. It was just a matter of personality.

Thanks to Javier, because of this experience, I felt sure that my future was in surgery, and not in primary care.

Chapter 7
A Large Baby

As the chief resident of the new Family Practice Program at Natividad Medical Center, I was responsible for many duties, even though I was just fresh out of my rotating internship at VMC. Both of these hospitals were affiliated with the medical school of the University of California San Francisco Medical Center.

I'd done a solid rotation in obstetrics in both medical school (at the Booth Memorial Hospital for unwed mothers in Omaha) and my internship, having delivered over 40 babies, but I was still wary of this department because I had seen how situations could change rapidly in a delivery. Even in experienced hands, things still could go wrong, and they did so in a matter of minutes.

The ob/gyn department at Natividad had only one staff, Dr. Lauderdale, who was the chief as well as the entire staff. He was a congenial man in his late fifties who had retired from the army at the nearby Fort Ord—now the home of the California State University, Monterey Bay—and began a second career. He spoke with a slight southern accent and I learned that he was originally from either North or South Carolina.

We got along well and he was a good teacher. The trouble was that he lived in Carmel, which was over an hour's drive away, and often there was dense fog that made the drive a great deal longer. My fear was that if I needed help, it would be difficult for him to get to the hospital in time.

Late one night, I was called in to the obstetrics ward. It was a beautiful November night, a little cool, and the moon was full, which made my walk from the apartment pleasant. As I headed to the labor room, my heart began racing. I had a foreboding feeling that this delivery might not go well, and Dr. Lauderdale wouldn't be able to get to the hospital in time.

The lighted clock on the wall read 1:20 am as I pushed open the doors of the ward, where I found a Hispanic woman in labor. She was a stout woman in her early forties who had delivered her previous five babies at Natividad. Maria Elena smiled and seemed happy to see me. Her husband, Jose, was in the waiting room, still in his work clothes. I learned that he worked as a mechanic at one of the lettuce farms, responsible for maintenance of the equipment that collected lettuce in the fields. Maria Elena also worked there as a picker.

Maria Elena spoke only a little English, and Jose spoke some as well. They looked like a lovely couple. She was a cooperative patient with a direct look in her hazel eyes. When she smiled, her eyes narrowed to crescents, revealing two gold teeth in the upper front.

Jose took his hat off and sat down in a chair, closing his eyes. It had probably been a busy day for him.

As I approached Maria Elena to examine her, I noticed that her strong, thick legs had bunches of large varicose veins about them like vines.

The nurse in charge reminded me that she was diabetic, and during the pregnancy her blood sugar hadn't been well controlled. Her blood pressure had been elevated and she was put on antihypertensive medications by Dr. Lauderdale. Both pieces of information only added to my worries because they were risk factors in the delivery. Diabetic women generally had large babies that often had more difficulty exiting the birth canal. The babies tended to be bigger because elevated sugar in the blood provided more calories for the fetus.

The nurse and I pushed Maria Elena from the labor room to the delivery room as her contractions grew stronger, and helped her transfer to the delivery table.

I examined her and found the baby's head high but the cervix fully dilated. Maria Elena had had many children, and her abdomen had become pendulous and lacked muscular tone, resulting in a slight misdirection of the forces of labor, which meant the baby's head was not situated in an optimal position.

I decided to monitor the baby with the fetal monitoring machine, thankful that I'd learned how to place the electrodes on the baby's scalp from my internship. When the machine started showing electrode signals, I began watching the monitor.

Maria Elena tried pushing, but her contractions weren't very strong and the baby wouldn't budge.

Realizing that it was a big baby, I worried that if it got stuck it would die, and perhaps endanger the mother's life as well. But with the obstetrician living an hour away, I knew I was Maria Elena and the baby's best chance.

Telling the woman to push harder, I was literally sweating and praying to God, "Please don't let this baby die." I enlarged the episiotomy.

An episiotomy is a surgical cut made at the opening of the vagina during childbirth, to aid a difficult delivery and prevent rupture of tissues.

I was fully aware of the possible complications of doing an episiotomy, such as lacerations into the anal sphincter.

The fetal monitor showed that the baby's heart rate was dropping, which was a sign of distress.

The most common causes of a slowing heart rate in the fetus include poor uterine perfusion, maternal hypotension, umbilical cord prolapse or occlusion, rapid fetal descent, placental abruption or uterine rupture, all of which would be disastrous to the baby and the mother.

It was a very bad sign. I had to get the baby out soon; otherwise, it would suffer anoxia and it might develop neurological deficits. Lack of oxygen was usually the cause of cerebral palsy.

The nurse told Maria Elena to push harder. She tried, but still the baby's head didn't move.

I had tried to call Dr. Lauderdale earlier, but there was no reply.

I tried to stay calm and went through the next steps in my mind. I thought about using the forceps to pull the baby's head out, but I'd never used them without supervision and I had witnessed how the use of them even in experienced hands still could do damage to the baby.

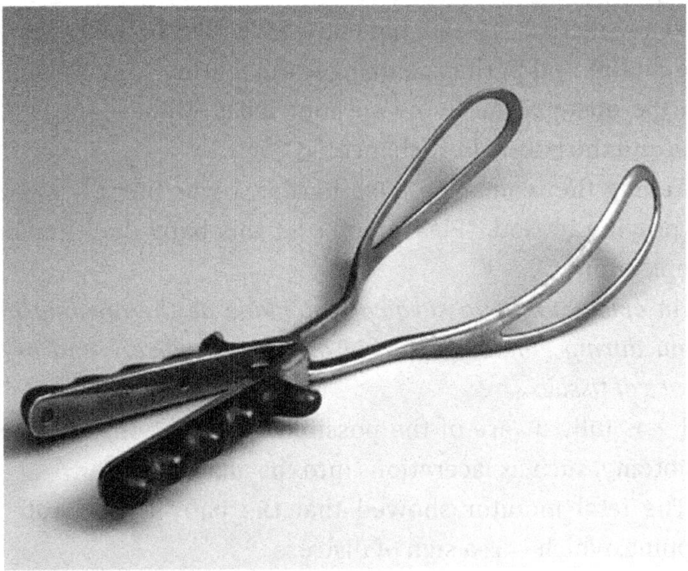

Delivery Forceps

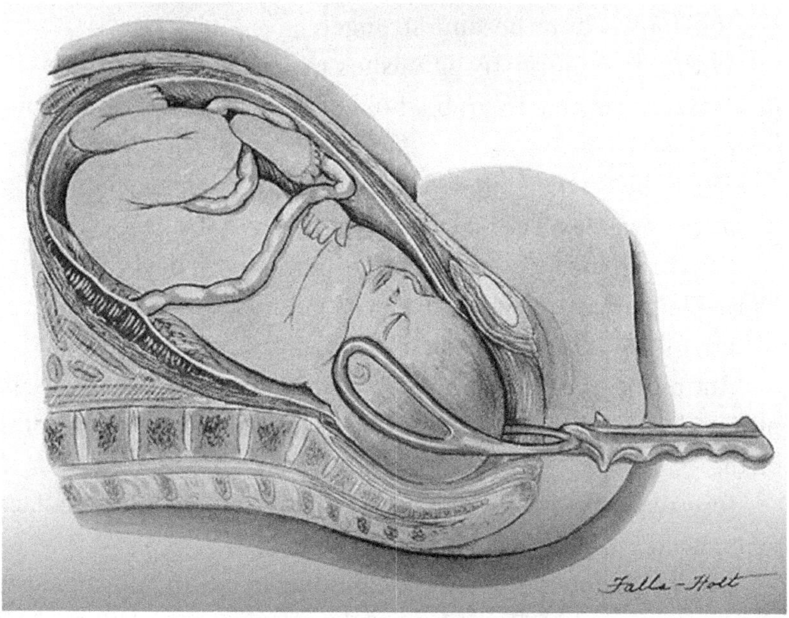

Forceps delivery of a baby

Now, the fetal monitor showed further slowing of the baby's heart rate. My own heart rate was increasing. I thought about the high malpractice judgments that had been awarded to injured babies, some of which were tens of millions of dollars. The highest one that came to mind was $100 million, which to me was simply absurd.

I tried not to think of it and concentrated on how to get the baby out.

I injected a little more Lidocaine to the area between the vagina and the rectum, and with the scissors, I enlarged the episiotomy further. I picked up two artery clamps and stopped the bleeding from the episiotomy.

I thought about giving Maria Elena Pitoxin to intensify the contractions. I was cautious since it was possible to cause a ruptured uterus where the muscles had been stretched by many pregnancies. So I gave her the minimal dose.

Her contractions became stronger.

With a few more strong pushes the baby's head dropped a little, and I was able to grab a hold of it with my hands and pull on it.

The baby finally exited. It was blue, but soon started crying. It was the sweetest cry I'd ever heard from a baby.

I tied the cord, cut it and lifted the baby, a boy, to hand to Maria Elena. He weighed over eleven pounds.

I thanked God for sparing us from a catastrophe!

Antibiotic eye ointment was placed in the baby's eyes to protect him from bacterial eye infections that can occur during birth.

Jose woke up from his nap and had a big smile on his face when he heard the news of his son's arrival.

I then sat down on the stool and began sewing up the large episiotomy as carefully as I could, because if it wasn't repaired correctly, fistulas could develop and lead to all sorts of complications. The fistulas would be much more difficult to repair later. When I was finished, the clock on the wall read 5 am.

Dr. Lauderdale finally responded to our page. I told him that the baby was delivered safely and it weighed almost twelve pounds. No wonder he had such a difficult time coming out.

With a big smile, Maria Elena told me that she would name her child Jaime, James in Spanish.

I hurried back to the apartment on the hospital grounds and tried to get a couple hours of sleep before my 8 am shift began at the general clinic.

That was the last delivery of my medical career. A few months later, I quit the family practice residency and switched to ophthalmology.

Chapter 8
Dolly

IT WAS A TUESDAY MORNING and things were beginning to get busy in the ER. The ambulance brought in a fifteen-year-old girl—who looked more like twenty—with shortness of breath and chest pain. From her history, I suspected it was pneumothorax, i.e. collapsed lung. I listened to her chest and found no breathing sounds on the right side.

The X-ray confirmed pneumothorax—her right lung was completely collapsed.

Since Dr. McCormick was now making it known that he was available for consultations, I presented the case to him, and he felt a chest tube was required. I'd put in a few chest tubes before and would have felt comfortable doing it, but since Dr. McCormick volunteered for it I was happy to leave the procedure to him—especially when I recalled a tragic incident in the ER just a month earlier.

Dr. Mike Berry, a staff physician, covered the ER from midnight till eight in the morning. In his mid-thirties, he and his wife and their three young children lived on a ranch. He and I got along well. He would report the conditions of the ER patients to me as I took over his shift in the morning.

In the nearby town Watsonville, a large Filipino population had come to the area to work on the farms a generation ago, and members of the community frequently utilized the hospital. Late one night an elderly Filipino couple showed up in the ER, the husband complaining of chest pain and difficulty breathing. Dr.

Berry took some chest X-rays and noted partial pneumothorax on one side.

The treatment was to insert a tube into the chest cavity, sucking the air out to re-inflate the collapsed lung. The procedure seemed brutal, because in order to put the plastic tube in the chest, a sharp instrument called a trochar—a metallic tube with a sharp triangular tip—had to be inserted along with the plastic tube. Once inside the chest cavity the trochar was withdrawn, leaving just the plastic tube, which was then connected to a constant suction, keeping the collapsed lung inflated.

The man was tiny, barely five feet tall, and extremely thin, with little connective tissue or fat. As Dr. Berry was pushing the trochar into the patient's chest cavity, the man let out a loud scream and went limp. Shortly afterward his blood pressure dropped to zero and he had no pulse. He had died. The sharp instrument had gone further than necessary, hitting the aorta, the large artery that carried blood from the heart to the rest of the body. He bled out quickly.

Hearing the scream, the patient's wife pulled the curtain aside and rushed in. Upon seeing her dead husband, she began wailing inconsolably and then suddenly collapsed. Resuscitation was attempted but failed. The couple had no children, only each other. She had died of a broken heart.

The local press heard about the incident—it was rumored that someone at the hospital tipped them off—and the next day the headlines claimed that Natividad hired incompetent doctors. Dr. Berry was a native of the area and had gone to medical school in Guadalajara, Mexico. The hospital conducted an inquiry and found that hitting the aorta with the trochar was one of the risks of the procedure. But they found fault with Dr. Berry in that the pneumo-thorax shown on the X-ray wasn't complete and the emergency placement of the chest tube was unnecessary—it could have waited. Mr. Santos, the eighty-five-year-old patient, could have been treated with oxygen until a specialist could be consulted in the morning.

In reality, at Natividad it wasn't easy to get consultations with specialists, and it often took days to get one. We did the best we could on the front line, but sometimes we weren't able to provide optimal care.

It's easy to speculate that such and such a step could have been taken to avoid the complication; but sometimes in medicine unpredictable things happen and patients die.

With that tragedy still fresh in my mind, I was more than happy to let Dr. McCormick put in Dolly's chest tube.

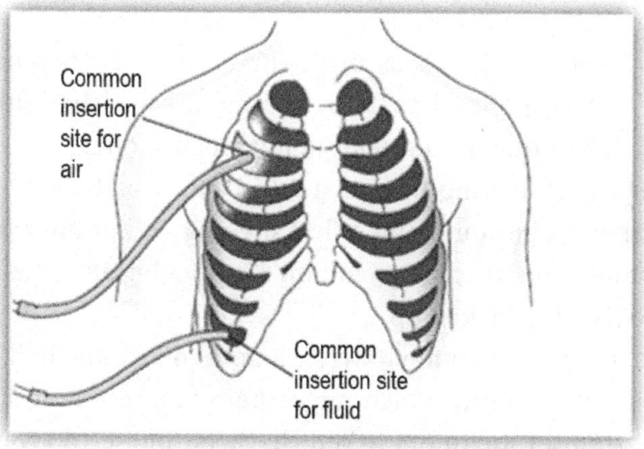

Placement of chest tubes

For pneumothorax, the tube is placed in the upper chest.
To drain fluid, the tube is placed in the lower chest.

The tube was inserted into Dolly's right chest without complication and was connected to a suction machine. The plan was to try to re-inflate the lung with suction, and most of the time this method worked. In some cases, when suction didn't work, surgery would be needed to seal the defect.

After the chest tube placement, Dolly was admitted to the hospital. I would see her twice a day, once early in the morning and then late in the afternoon. In addition, I was always on call for her.

The next morning when I visited Dolly, her mother was there.

"Dr. Hung, please take good care of Dolly," Mrs. Hurley pleaded. "She's my baby and my only child."

"Of course I will," I responded with a nod.

I listened to Dolly's chest, which still had no breathing sounds on the right. But she was comfortable and no longer had any pain or shortness of breath. I checked the entry wound of the chest tube, and it showed no signs of infection. She didn't have a fever. All the cases of pneumothorax I'd taken care of before had responded to this treatment, and their lungs re-inflated in less than two weeks, many much sooner.

In spite of looking like an adult, Dolly was behaving like a five-year-old. She complained that she missed her boyfriend, but her mother told her Roy couldn't come because he was in juvenile hall, i.e., locked up.

Mrs. Hurley asked me to write a note to juvenile hall to see if Roy could visit Dolly, which might help her recover faster. Not willing to upset anyone, I asked the head nurse to type up the note, which was promptly done, and then I signed it.

Two days later, Roy did visit Dolly, along with a sheriff. I happened to show up just as Roy and the sheriff were leaving. Roy had chains around his ankles and tattoos all over his body, including his forehead. I couldn't understand how a fifteen-year-old girl could have such boyfriend.

I didn't look forward to checking on Dolly during my rounds, as her childish behavior was annoying; but I tried my best to be attentive and respond to her and her mother's questions and requests.

Two weeks went by and Dolly's lung remained collapsed. Dr. McCormick was nowhere to be found and his pager went unanswered.

Then rumors had been circulating that Dr. McCormick had a drinking problem. Initially, I refused to believe it.

Four weeks went by, Dolly's lung remained collapsed, and there was still no sign of the doctor.

One evening the nurse from the ward called to tell me that Dolly was shivering and had a high fever. I rushed to the hospital and found Dolly's mother crying, saying her daughter was going to die.

I examined Dolly, concluding that she'd developed sepsis, and immediately started her on IV antibiotics. Soon she stopped shivering and her temperature returned to normal. Dolly's mother had been partially right—if left untreated, the sepsis could've killed her.

The blood culture showed that the combination antibiotics were the correct drugs for the infection, which I suspected was most likely caused by the prolonged use of the chest tube.

By now it had been almost six weeks since Dolly's chest tube had been placed. I consulted the other staff physicians, including the director of the hospital, but no one could offer me any suggestions as to what I should do. We'd given the chest tube enough time and it wasn't working, and now Dolly needed surgery. I was still a resident and should have backup help, but no help was available.

Dolly's mother was furious with the hospital, but she understood my predicament and wasn't angry with me—although she certainly would've been if her daughter had died! Realizing that her daughter needed surgery, Mrs. Hurley was able to talk the only other thoracic and vascular surgeon in town into taking over Dolly's care, asking me to be in the ambulance during Dolly's transfer to the private hospital.

Two days later I was the first assistant to Dr. Cibis, a huge German with red hair, who took out the infected chest tube, opened the chest and rubbed talcum powder (sterile baby power) into the defect in the chest wall to cause the inflammation and scar tissue formation that would seal the leak. The surgery worked and Dolly's right lung re-inflated.

Dolly could have died and I would have been responsible, because I was indeed her physician, even though I wasn't qualified to take care of such a patient without supervision. After all, I was still a resident in training.

It was a close call. Dr. McCormick never showed up at the hospital again and I was convinced that the rumors were true and he had an alcohol problem.

I cannot imagine what I would have done if Dolly had died.

Chapter 9
The Family from Vietnam

The Fall of Saigon, also known as the Liberation of Saigon by North Vietnamese, was the capture of Saigon, the capital of South Vietnam, by the People's Army of Vietnam and the Viet Cong on April 30, 1975.

SAIGON HAD FALLEN to the communists and many Vietnamese were risking their lives to leave their country. Four members of an extended Chinese Vietnamese family had settled in Salinas. The man, Tran—which I later learned was Chen in Chinese—in his early thirties, his wife Minh, his sister Binh and his wife's teenage brother, Jimmy Nguyen, had boarded a less-than-seaworthy boat crowded with refugees, trying to find someplace to land.

During the many days at sea, some of the refugees died and were simply thrown overboard, because there was no other way to deal with the bodies. The boat made it to the east coast of peninsular Malaya in Malaysia, not far from Kota Baharu. But they were met with hostility from the mostly Muslim Malays in the area. Some refugees from Vietnam had made it to Malaysia earlier, but most Malays didn't want any more of them. So, the boat was pushed back out to sea. Unable to land, they had no choice but to continue their search for a safe place.

Eventually the boat made it to Hong Kong, where the family was confined to a refugee camp for seven months. Conditions in Hong Kong were difficult, as they were treated like prisoners, confined to tiny quarters and not allowed to leave the camp. An NGO finally connected the family with a church group in

Minnesota, which sponsored them to come to America. Unable to stand the severe cold in Minnesota, they eventually found their way to Salinas, after learning from a relative that they could find work in the area's many lettuce fields.

When the family showed up at the ER, none of them knew more than a few words of English and I was called to act as interpreter—they spoke a provincial Cantonese with a Vietnamese accent. They were at Natividad because Tran's wife Minh was pregnant.

They all looked scared. Tran was a slim man of about five feet five inches, with hollow cheeks and dry, lifeless hair. Minh was a petite woman with a shy smile, no taller than five feet, who looked quite pregnant. Tran's sister Binh looked like her brother, with the same hollow cheeks. Minh's brother Jimmy Nguyen looked about fourteen—he had a round face like his sister, and he spoke the most English. But he seemed embarrassed and wasn't willing to interpret for the family, claiming that he only spoke a little English.

Dr. Lauderdale was going to examine Minh and asked me to help with communication. He estimated that Minh was about eight months into her pregnancy. I went over his instructions with Tran and Minh, and also gave them a supply of prenatal vitamins. We ran some tests to assess Minh's hemoglobin as well as her kidney function.

I learned that the family didn't have a car and the public transportation in Salinas was non-existent—they had walked to the hospital from downtown. At the end of the examination and instructions, I told them that if they didn't mind waiting, I would take them back home when I finished my shift at the ER.

My replacement came in at 5 pm, and the entire family got into my small gray hatchback Ford Mustang.

They had a small apartment on the second floor of an old building in the worst part of downtown Salinas, surrounded by men holding bottles in brown paper bags.

As they were getting out of the car, I told Minh to be sure to take her vitamins daily and to come back in for a check-up in a month.

I stayed in the car and watched them walk up to their dilapidated apartment. I imagined what they'd gone through, being turned away in Malaysia, and now, even in the country of so many people's dreams, their life wasn't at all easy. They didn't know the language. They had little money and they didn't appear to be educated.

When Minh failed to show up for her return appointment I became concerned, noticing that the due date on her chart was very close. The family didn't have a phone for me to contact them, so I decided to make a house call. After my shift at the hospital ER, I headed for downtown.

This part of Salinas was unfamiliar to me. Men sat around drinking, some quite obviously drunk. Some of them were talking loudly, and others were singing in Spanish. I found the building and parked my car in front of it.

I smiled and waved to two men sitting by the stairs, laughing loudly, each holding a bottle in a brown paper bag. They smiled and waved back.

Walking up the stairs and knocking at the door, I was relieved when Minh answered. She was home alone; her husband and sister-in-law were working in a Chinese restaurant nearby and Jimmy was at school. She seemed frightened and told me that earlier in the day she began leaking fluid, not understanding that she'd ruptured her membranes and it was an emergency. Once the membranes are ruptured, the baby needs to be delivered or it will die.

I explained to her the urgency of getting her to the hospital right away.

I left a note in English for her brother Jimmy and one in Chinese for her husband, to let them know that I'd taken Minh to the hospital for delivery.

That evening, Dr. Lauderdale started Minh on a Pitoxin drip to induce labor. I was assigned to the ER, and was there mainly as an interpreter. Soon her contractions started, and an hour later she delivered a healthy boy weighing just under seven pounds.

"Jim, I can't imagine what would've happened to this baby boy if you hadn't gone to Mrs. Tran's to check up on her," remarked Dr. Lauderdale.

"We were lucky," I replied.

"Without sufficient amniotic fluid, a baby is at risk of suffering serious health complications," he added. "I can't imagine how this poor family would deal with a baby with those kinds of problems."

The rest of the family showed up later in the evening, and everyone was overjoyed. A son was very important for Chinese and Vietnamese families.

It was the best deed I did during my time at Natividad. I felt that destiny had brought us together. The Trans knew that if I hadn't shown up at their apartment that day, the baby would most certainly have died that evening or the following day. I was so thankful that I was able to do something good, a deed that meant so much to the family and yet at little expense on my behalf—only the very minor inconvenience of checking on Minh at the apartment. It was good karma.

I wish I'd kept in touch with the family after I left Natividad. There was no doubt in my mind that they would do well, and they're probably living comfortably somewhere in California.

The boy whose life I saved would be about forty-eight years old now, and would certainly have a family of his own.

Chapter 10

Too Young to Die

IN THE SPRING OF 1976, we were packing and getting ready to embark on the next segment of our life journey.

I hadn't taken a rotation in ophthalmology in medical school, so I was planning to spend a few months at the New York Eye and Ear Infirmary to get some experience in ophthalmology before I began my residency on July 1.

My nine months at Natividad had been trying, but I think, in the end, they were very beneficial. I had gained so much more experience and knowledge in general medicine, and I was confident taking care of almost anything that came into the ER. I had learned various life-saving procedures such as putting in chest tubes, inserting a central line in the sub-clavian vein, putting tubes in people's tracheas and the burr hole procedure, which I wouldn't hesitate to do if a patient came in with a subdural hematoma and there wasn't a neurosurgeon around.

Mary would be going home to Michigan with our daughter Melissa, and they would travel to the East Coast with her mother to visit her sister.

I had reserved a room at the Gramercy Park Hotel at 2 Lexington Ave, in lower Manhattan, two blocks from the eye hospital.

We were excited about this next stage of our lives. I was relieved that after hesitating among several specialties, including psychiatry, pediatrics, family practice, urology and orthopedics, I finally settled on ophthalmology.

As we prepared to leave, my work at Natividad was still extremely busy. But by now I was getting paid over $5,000 a month, which I considered a great deal of money.

I read in the paper that a donut shop in Salinas had an outbreak of hepatitis A. Initially, a couple—the shop owners—got sick, but soon all six of their employees got sick too.

Hepatitis means inflammation of the liver. The liver is a vital organ that processes nutrients, filters the blood and fights infections. When the liver is inflamed or damaged, its function can be affected.

The donut shop owners and staff all showed up at the general clinic in Natividad for evaluation. All of them tested positive for hepatitis A. Most of them were feeling fine, with the exception of two young women.

One was hospitalized for a few days and then was well enough to be discharged and sent home. At the time, there was really no specific treatment for hepatitis. Some claimed prednisone was beneficial in reducing the amount of damage to the liver, but there were no good studies to prove it.

Another young woman, a nineteen-year-old Hartnell College student who worked part time at the donut shop, did not improve. Her conjunctiva was obviously yellow, indicating jaundice and liver damage.

Amy was a slim, attractive brunette with short hair and large brown eyes. She was taking some science classes at college with the hope of going into nursing.

When I initially examined Amy, she had a fever and seemed tired, and she said she had no appetite. Because of her inability to take any food, I decided to keep her in the hospital longer.

I followed her closely with daily liver enzyme studies, which alarmingly showed progressive worsening of her liver.

Her parents were extremely concerned as asked me what I thought of Amy's prognosis. I said it was difficult to tell, but that from my experience, most people recovered from such an infection.

Concerned that Amy was getting worse and that I might be missing something, I called the liver specialist at Stanford University and asked for advice. He said there was really not much we could do for patients with hepatitis and reassured me that most hepatitis A patients would recover.

***

In rare cases, hepatitis A can cause liver failure and even death; this is more common in older people and in those with other serious health issues, such as chronic liver disease.

Mild cases resolve without any permanent liver damage. It's rare for healthy adults to die from hepatitis A, and the illness doesn't become chronic.

While I was reading about the disease, I also learned that there are several types of hepatitis.

Hepatitis A: This type won't lead to long-term infection and usually doesn't cause any complications. Most people heal in about two months, and it can be prevented with a vaccine.

The main way we get hepatitis A is by eating or drinking something that has the hepatitis A virus in it. A lot of times this happens in a restaurant. If an infected worker there doesn't wash their hands well after using the bathroom, and then touches food, they could pass the disease to another person.

It's also a sexually transmitted infection (STI) passed on through unprotected sexual activities.

Hepatitis B: Most people recover from this type in six months. Sometimes, though, it causes a long-term infection that could lead to liver damage. Once a person gets the disease, he or she can spread the virus even if there are no symptoms.

A minority of people may develop severe symptoms during an acute hepatitis B infection, and in rare cases it can lead to death. After the acute stage (more than six months after infection), many people with chronic hepatitis B have few or no symptoms.

The hepatitis B virus can be spread in the following ways: unprotected sex; living in a household with a person with chronic (life-long) HBV infection; and sharing personal care items such as toothbrushes, razors or nail clippers.

Hepatitis C: Many people with this type don't have symptoms. About 80% of those with the disease get a long-term infection, i.e., a chronic infection, which may lead to cirrhosis.

The hepatitis C virus is usually spread when someone comes into contact with blood from an infected person, such as through a blood transfusion.

Today, most people become infected with hepatitis C by sharing needles, syringes or any other equipment used to prepare and inject drugs

***

Amy was placed in an isolation room, and anyone going into her room had to wear a gown and gloves, as hepatitis A was very infectious.

As her physician, I was in close contact with her daily.

She was getting progressively weaker and complained that she felt really bad and was uncomfortable no matter how she lay in bed.

One morning, I noted bleeding from her nose. (A damaged liver cannot produce the chemicals that help the blood to clot.) The same afternoon, it looked like she had a stroke and she became unresponsive. I consulted the head of the hospital and he suggested that Amy be intubated.

I requested a neurology consultation to assess the status of her brain activity. The neurologist was quite sure that she had bleeding in her brain, just as she was bleeding from her nose.

At the time, I was barely thirty years old, with a wife and a two-year-old daughter. I was petrified that I would end up like Amy. But there was no way of abandoning her care because I had admitted her to the hospital and she was my patient from the beginning.

The bleeding from her nose became more profuse. I had to suction the blood, and I cleaned her endotracheal tube as well. By now, she was totally unresponsive. I would prick her leg with a safety pin, and there would be no reaction.

I tried to be as careful as I could, wearing two masks when I went into her room. But the specter of her lying in bed motionlessly really bothered me. She wasn't even twenty. How was it possible that this young woman, who three weeks ago was active and full of life, going to school, trying to become a nurse, now no longer had any life in her motionless body? She was just beginning to live her life. And she got this virus while trying to make a few dollars at a donut shop. I thought it was so unfair.

When I got home at night, I stood under the shower for half an hour, trying to wash any bit of virus from my body. I didn't want to spread it to Mary or Melissa.

Soon Amy's kidneys also began to fail. Her face became puffy and swollen, quite different from the pretty woman who had first arrived at the hospital. Before long, her legs were swollen as well.

I called the liver specialist at Stanford again, and he again told me that there was nothing he could do, and there was no reason for me to transfer Amy to his hospital. He added that it was very unusual for someone with hepatitis A to be in this condition.

Next, I called the nephrologist. He came and evaluated Amy's kidneys and indicated that without hemodialysis, Amy wouldn't last more than a few days.

When Amy's parents arrived later, I explained the situation to them.

"What's the point of dialysis if her brain is gone?" asked Amy's mother.

"I agree with you," I responded. "I'll have a meeting with the other doctors."

At a loss for what to do, I insisted on having a meeting with as many staff physicians as I could to discuss what we should do about Amy.

One physician suggested that Amy be re-evaluated by the neurologist to check if there was any brain activity.

The EEG was done, and it showed that Amy was brain dead. It was difficult to relate the information to Amy's parents. I showed them the neurologist's evaluation and explained that Amy had no brain activity.

Her parents were grief-stricken, but told me to do whatever I thought was appropriate, understanding that it was extremely unlikely Amy would regain any brain function.

I again talked to the head of the hospital to update him on Amy's condition, saying that her parents were ready for us to stop the ventilator that was keeping her alive. I insisted that he write a note on her chart indicating his agreement that further heroic treatment would be futile. The neurologist, too, wrote a long note, explaining his findings and giving his opinion that there was no way Amy would recover and further treatment would only prolong her death.

It was a Sunday morning. The sun was shining brightly in the beautiful Salinas Valley. Amy's parents were in the room, and the minister from their church was present. We watched Amy's lifeless body and the ventilator causing her chest to rise and fall.

"Are you ready?" I asked Amy's parents.

They nodded.

I turned off the ventilator machine and we watched Amy. There was no response, not a sound, not even a slight movement. Without the ventilator, Amy died a peaceful death.

Amy's death raised many questions in my mind. It bothered me that there was nothing we could do for this young woman. I pondered life, why some die so young, while others live to a hundred. The mystery of life just became more mysterious to me.

Life is so unfair.

Chapter 11

Willie Walker

IT WAS DECEMBER OF 1976, just a few months into the first year of my ophthalmology residency, when I met Willie Walker. He was a handsome, 40-year-old Black American, over six feet tall with strong arms, a good physique and a big smile.

His clinical records, which consisted of three volumes, was over six inches thick. He'd been a patient at the clinic since he was six years old. I learned that during the previous decade, most of his clinic visits were more social than medical, as when I first saw him, he was almost completely blind and there was nothing we could do for him at that point. Not only was he almost completely blind, able to see shadows only, but he was also almost completely deaf.

I went through his medical records from the beginning, noting that his vision was 20/60 in each eye when he was first seen. Over the years, his vision got worse and worse. When he was old enough to take a visual field test, it showed progressive visual field loss in each eye. Now, he only had a very small island of vision.

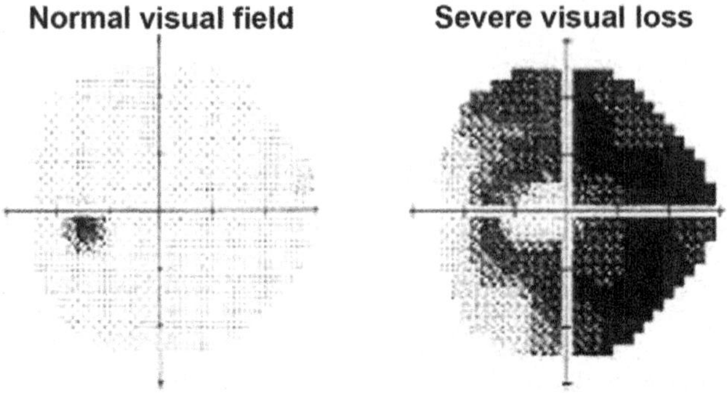

A small island of vision, i.e., tunnel vision

The day I met Willie, he showed up at the clinic by himself. We struck up a friendship and I tried to learn as much as I could about his life.

At that point, it was very difficult to communicate with him because he was essentially blind and deaf. He could still hear just a little, although his hearing aid didn't help much. The only way I could communicate with him was through touching and writing on his palm. I had tried talking loudly into his ears, but that didn't seem to help, and it only added confusion to the busy clinic. But he was able to talk, since he had adequate hearing growing up and had learned to speak normally, unlike those born completely deaf who never heard the tones of speech, and were thus unable to learn how to speak properly.

As Willie and I figured out how to communicate, he asked, "Are you excited that Jimmy Carter will be our new president?"

"He is a good man," I replied.

He agreed and seemed truly excited about the new president.

I learned that Willie lived in West Fresno with his parents. There was no history of blindness or deafness in his family and both his parents had normal hearing and eyesight. When he was six years old, it became evident that he had a hearing problem. He was evaluated by an audiologist who confirmed that he did indeed have hearing loss. He was seen by his pediatrician who made the diagnosis of Usher syndrome.

Willie attended a school for the deaf for years, and learned sign language. But as he got older, he began to complain more about his vision.

Even though his pediatrician had already made the diagnosis of Usher syndrome, he was sent to the eye clinic at UCSF Medical Center for further diagnostic tests to confirm that he had the eye problem that went along with Usher syndrome.

Willie got the equivalent of a high school diploma, but he couldn't find a suitable job. He told me that he had many hobbies, one of which was short wave ham radio, and he made friends all over the world. He told me that he'd talked with a blind jazz guitar player in New Orleans for years. He also talked to someone in the Outback of Australia, but he said the fellow's accent was so strong that it was difficult to understand all of what he said. But with his hearing getting bad, talking over the ham radio was getting more difficult.

I was amazed by Willie's optimism. After our first encounter, I wondered about his life. How did he manage to take the bus when he was now almost completely blind and deaf? How did he cross the street? How did he know which direction to go after he got off the bus?

When he left, I read up on Usher syndrome, and I've since learned new things about it beyond what I knew in 1976.

Usher syndrome is the most common condition that affects both hearing and vision, and it can even affect balance. The major symptoms are hearing loss or deafness, and a degeneration of the retina called *retinitis pigmentosa* (RP).

The hearing loss is caused by the abnormal development of hair cells (sound receptors) in the inner ear. Moderate to profound hearing loss is usually present at birth, but occasionally hearing loss associated with Usher syndrome appears in adolescence or later.

Balance problems can also occur through the abnormal development of vestibular hair cells—sensory cells that detect gravity and head movement. When I read about it, I was so glad Willie didn't have any balance problems—it would have really restricted his movements.

Retinitis Pigmentosa (RP) initially causes night-blindness and a gradual loss of peripheral (side) vision resulting from the progressive degeneration of cells in the retina. The retina is the light-sensitive tissue at the back of the eye, crucial for vision. As RP progresses, the field of vision narrows until eventually only central vision—or tunnel vision—remains.

The syndrome is inherited, passed from parents to children genetically. Each child inherits a gene from each parent, and if one or more of the genes is mutated, cells may develop or act abnormally.

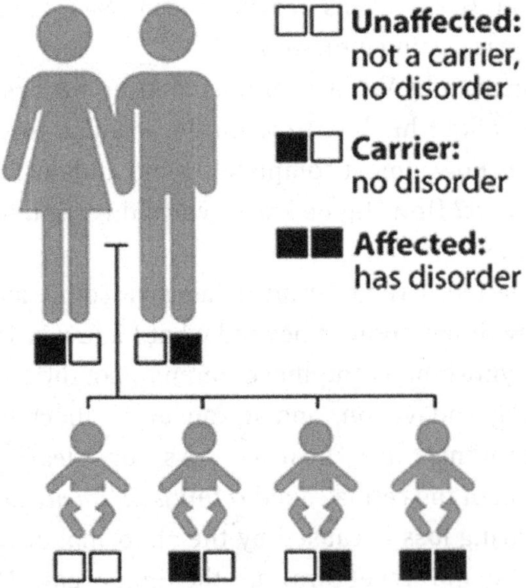

Autosomal recessive inheritance

Usher syndrome is inherited as an autosomal recessive disorder. "Autosomal" means that both men and women are equally likely to have a particular trait or condition, and equally likely to pass it down to a child of either sex. "Recessive" means that the disorder only occurs when a child inherits two copies of the same faulty gene, one from each parent. Someone with one abnormal Usher gene doesn't have the disorder—but they become a carrier, with a 50% chance of passing the abnormal gene to their children. If two carriers of the same mutated gene have children, each child has a:

- One-in-four chance of having a child who neither has Usher syndrome nor is a carrier.
- Two-in-four chance of having a child who is an unaffected carrier.
- One-in-four chance of having a child who has Usher syndrome.

I also read further about the three types of Usher syndrome. In the United States, types 1 and 2 are the most common, accounting for up to 95% of cases combined.

Type 1: Children with type 1 Usher syndrome have profound hearing loss or deafness at birth and severe balance problems. There's often little or no benefit to fitting them with hearing aids, but nowadays they may be candidates for a cochlear implant—an electronic device that gives a sense of sound to a deaf or severely hard-of-hearing person.

Balance problems in type 1 Usher syndrome babies cause a delay in sitting up without support, and walking rarely occurs before 18 months.

Vision problems usually appear before age 10, starting with difficulty seeing at night and progressing to severe vision loss over several decades.

Type 2: Children with type 2 Usher syndrome are born with moderate to severe hearing loss, but have normal balance. The severity of hearing loss varies, but most children with type 2 Usher syndrome develop normal speech and can benefit from hearing aids. RP is usually diagnosed during late adolescence in people with type 2 Usher syndrome.

Type 3: Children with type 3 Usher syndrome are born with normal hearing. Most of them have normal or near-normal balance, but some develop balance problems as they age. The decline in hearing and vision can vary. Hearing loss often materializes by adolescence, and hearing aids are required by mid to late adulthood. Night blindness usually appears in adolescence as well, with blind spots developing by the late teens or early twenties. Legal blindness often occurs by mid-life.

When Willie was a patient at the clinic, it was long before the days of genetic testing. Now genetic testing may help in diagnosing Usher syndrome. So far, researchers have found nine genes that cause Usher syndrome. Genetic testing is available for all of them:

- Type 1 Usher syndrome: *MY07A, USH1C, CDH23, PCHD15, USH1G*
- Type 2 Usher syndrome: *USH2A, GPR98, DFNB31*
- Type 3 Usher syndrome: *CLRN1*

Currently, there's no known cure for Usher syndrome. Treatment involves the management of hearing, vision and balance issues. An early diagnosis can help educators develop programs that accommodate the issues facing children with the syndrome. Communication aids and education can include hearing aids, listening devices, cochlear implants, auditory training and sign language lessons. Later, independent-living training can help Usher syndrome patients with orientation and mobility for balance issues, Braille instruction and low-vision services.

A study conducted by the National Eye Institute and the Foundation Fighting Blindness found that Vitamin A may slow the progression of RP.

Willie's case wasn't clear-cut, but he seemed to have the type 2 variety.

When Willie returned in six months, he was as cheerful as before. It was now June and getting hot in Fresno.

His head was soaked with sweat. He'd taken the bus from his house, and had to walk the last half mile to the clinic.

"I don't mind the heat," he remarked. "I was born here and I'm used to it."

"What have you been doing?" I asked.

"I've kept busy," he replied. "I help my mother with her garden. We planted tomatoes, okra, green beans and eggplants. I also help her collect eggs from the chicken coop each morning. I exercise regularly, and my favorite thing to do is chin-ups. I can do twenty in a row," he said with a wide grin.

"If I get really bored at home, I take the bus and ride around town, even though I can't see," he continued. "All the bus drivers know me, and they're all very nice to me. Most of them are happy to see me. Many of them shake my hand and pat me on my shoulder as I get on the bus. I know all their names. Some of them even forget I can't hear sometimes and try to talk to me.

"I know they're not supposed to talk to me while they're driving, but I think many of them get lonely driving the bus all day long," he laughed.

"Sometimes early in the morning, I walk to the Fresno Zoo and sit on a bench. When I was a boy, my mama used to take me there every week. Now, I can still remember where the different animals are. The zoo brings back a lot of good memories," he added.

"You are truly amazing," I tried to tell him by writing on his palm.

He smiled. "Most people are very nice to me. I have this notebook that I hang around my neck, and if I really need help, I show the book to someone—it says I'm blind and deaf. I especially need help when I cross the street because I can't hear the traffic. When there's no one around, I raise my red and white cane as high as I can, and wave it up and down so people can see me."

Willie again returned six months later. Now the weather was cool again.

"I like this cool weather much better," he remarked.

I held his right palm and wrote in it that I was very happy to see him, and he gave me a big smile.

"I have a girlfriend," he announced.

"Tell me more," I wrote in his palm.

"She's a hairdresser in the neighborhood," he said. "She's really nice. My favorite thing is to eat at the Popeye Fried Chicken place with her. She treats me really nice," he added.

It looked like Willie was in love, because he seemed even happier than his usual self, beaming widely.

"I am so happy for you," I wrote in his palm.

I always looked forward to visiting with Willie, even though we both knew there was nothing we could do for his eyesight.

He wanted to keep returning, because if there were any new developments in the treatment of the disease, he wanted to know.

I often think of Willie. The human spirit is resilient. Willie made the best of his situation and tried to live as happy a life as he could.

At times, when I've felt low or things haven't gone my way, I've reminded myself of Willie.

Sometimes we can learn so much about life from our patients. It was the luck of the draw. It just happened that both of Willie's parents carried a very rare recessive gene and he ended up having this debilitating condition. But he seemed to be a happier person than many others who had everything by comparison.

After I returned from my fellowship in retina surgery and opened my own private practice, I saw Willie on several occasions while I was driving, walking with his cane in different parts of town.

He really got around. His handicap never stopped him from living a full life.

Chapter 12

Shorty

AT THE BEGINNING OF 1977, I was halfway into the first year of my three-year ophthalmology residency. In the first year, the new residents would see clinic patients and take care of all the minor problems, such as infections. We also began to learn about strabismus—deviation of the eye, found almost always in children—and learn how to do surgery to correct it.

I assisted in the senior resident's surgeries, although we often simply observed. After half a year, the first-year residents were given an opportunity to play with the operating microscope. Learning to operate under the microscope was a tricky thing, as we had to learn new hand-eye coordination. Since the operating microscope made the object larger, we had to adjust to the new spatial relationship, such as how much movement to make, how to use the micro scissors, and how to put a suture on the eye.

It took me several months just to learn how to use it; then, toward the end of my first year, I was allowed to begin doing surgeries on patients with pterygium.

Pterygium is a noncancerous, triangular growth that may occur on one or both eyes. It's more common in people with darker pigment who spend a lot of time in the sun, such as those who work outdoors.

The painless growth may be slightly raised and contain obvious blood vessels. It may cause irritation and possibly affect vision. In severe cases, surgery may be necessary.

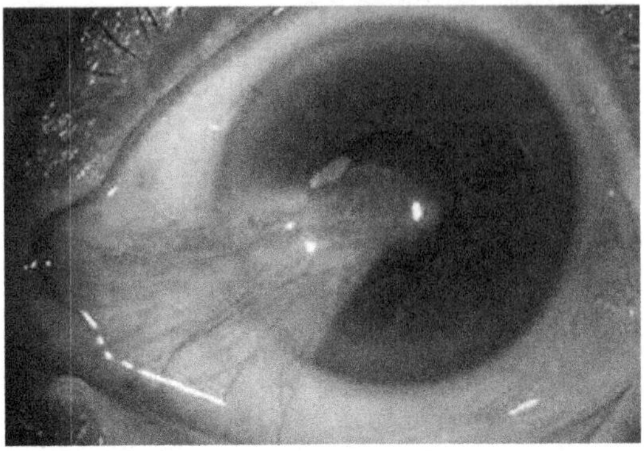

A pterygium

I had already done over ten such surgeries and all of them had gone well. The surgery to remove the pterygium was the ideal procedure for the first-year residents, as we could see the lesion very clearly under the microscope, and the cornea is actually a very tough tissue that would be difficult to damage. Of course, the danger of cutting too deep was always present, but we could always see the depth of the blade clearly under the operating microscope.

Shorty's real name was Julio Martinez, but I could see why he had the nickname. He was less than five feet tall, stocky, with a potbelly. His round head was covered in dense, wavy, dark brown hair, and he wore a small mustache. Because of the wrinkles on his very tanned, weather-beaten face, he looked older than the fifty years I'd noted on his chart.

He worked on a farm in Reedley, a town some twenty miles from Fresno. He spoke almost no English, but his younger brother, who looked like a younger version of Shorty, was friendly and loquacious and spoke decent English. Augustus, who went by Gus, explained to me that his father named him because he was born in August, whereas Shorty was born in July and hence his name, Julio. Gus worked as a foreman on the same farm as his brother.

Shorty was in the clinic because of irritation in both eyes caused by inflamed pterygia, and in his left eye, the growth was now blocking his vision.

I examined Shorty and found two very irritated eyes, beefy red and swollen.

It was obvious that Shorty needed surgery in his left eye, as the growth had reached his pupillary area. In order to get the best outcome, we generally wanted to quiet down the inflammation first with a course of prednisone eye drops.

When Shorty returned in two weeks, both eyes were no longer inflamed. He was scheduled for surgery the following Thursday, our usual surgery day.

Under the operating microscope, I carefully dissected the growth on his cornea and peeled it free. I then carefully removed the entire growth. The conjunctiva was then tagged down by suturing it to the sclera with two absorbable sutures, a little distance from the cornea.

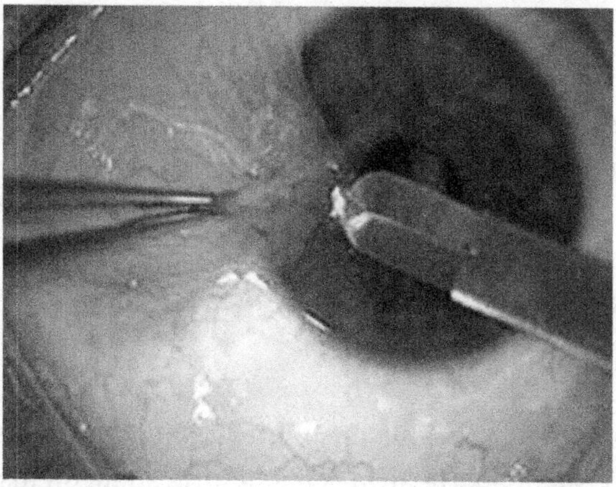

Pterygium surgery under the microscope

We had learned that we should use as little cautery as possible, as the charring of the tissue could exacerbate a recurrence, in some groups as high as fifty percent. At the end of the procedure, I was satisfied with the results. I applied a prednisone-antibiotic combination ointment in Shorty's eye and patched it, and asked him to return the following day.

The next day, there was no sign of infection and Shorty seemed comfortable. I handed Gus two prescriptions, one for *Maxitrol,* a prednisone-antibiotic combination drop, and the second for *Thiotepa,* with instructions for Shorty to instill in his left eye three times a day, alternating the two drops, while awake.

Shorty belonged to the group with a high recurrence rate because of his heavy pigment, and also because of his working environment—dusty, hot and exposed to the sunlight much of the time—which was the reason I prescribed Thiotepa, as I'd done with my other Latino, black and some Asian patients.

The custom in the clinic was to use a drug after surgery to discourage fast healing, which was thought to be the cause of most recurrence. In this group of patients, we generally used Thiotepa, a radiomimetic drug that inhibits rapidly proliferating cells.

Thiotepa is related chemically and pharmacologically to the nitrogen mustards, and having a radiomimetic effect, was developed to be used systematically for the treatment of certain neoplastic diseases.

Beta irradiation had also been used by ophthalmic surgeons for many years.

During our three previous encounters, Shorty rarely spoke. He was a very shy man. He always had a little smile on his face, and always avoided eye contact with me. Gus did all the talking for him.

I explained to him through Gus that one drop was to prevent recurrence and the other was to reduce inflammation and prevent infection.

He was to return in a week.

The following Friday, when I examined him with the slit lamp, I almost fell off my stool. Instead of healing slowly, the wound had deepened and there was a depression in the cornea and sclera. My heart jumped into my mouth. My immediate thought was that Shorty was going to lose his eye, because not only was the wound not healing, it had actually gotten worse. And if it deepened further, it would develop into a hole and the eye would be lost.

I immediately summoned the senior resident, who was also surprised to see the non-healing wound. It happened that the chairman of the department was in his office, and he too examined Shorty. We were all scratching our heads. I'd done at least ten such operations before, and nothing like this had ever happened.

The three of us left the examination room and went to the chairman's office.

"What should we do?" I asked.

"We have to find out why the wound isn't healing," said the chairman. "I saw a similar case when I was in training. The radiologist gave the patient too large a dose of beta irradiation, which caused the wound not to heal. The patient needed a conjunctiva flap from another area to cover the wound, and it finally healed."

A light bulb suddenly went off in my head, and I rushed back to the examination room and asked Shorty to show me his eye drops. I looked at the Thiotepa bottle carefully, and my heart sank.

Instead of a 1:2000 solution of Thiotepa, it was 1:200—ten times the strength it was supposed to be.

I called the pharmacy and asked them to check on my original prescription. It was faxed to the chairman's office, and it showed, in my handwriting, that I had prescribed 1:200 instead of 1:2000. I had neglected one zero.

Now we knew it was the Thiotepa that had caused the tissue not to heal.

The chairman suggested that I patch the eye and check Shorty daily. If it got worse, a conjunctival flap should be considered. A conjunctival flap would move the conjunctiva from another area to cover the defect.

I returned to the examination room and faced the music.

"Lo siento," I said to Shorty. He looked at me, puzzled.

"Gus," I said, "please tell your brother that I am very sorry. I gave him a stronger eye drop and it's not healing well. I need to patch his eye and see him tomorrow."

Shorty seemed confused but remained quiet.

It was lunchtime, but I had lost my appetite. I was feeling very bad that I'd caused this disaster. I walked out of the clinic into the hospital's courtyard and sat under a tree, saying some prayers and asking God to please let Shorty heal.

I'd been fortunate that none of my patients died during my internship or the year of my family practice residency because of my negligence, ignorance or sloth.

Now, because of my negligence, I might have caused a patient to lose his eye.

Many thoughts ran through my mind. I remembered the story about an ophthalmologist who removed the wrong eye (the good one instead of the one filled with cancer), and he ended up killing himself because he felt so bad. That disaster happened because of a series of mistakes made by the nursing staff on the floor, the orderly and the surgical nurse who had marked the wrong eye. The doctor himself erred by not asking the patient himself which eye before the anesthesiologist put him to sleep. It wouldn't have happened if any one of the mistakes had been caught.

I also recalled when, just a year ago, a senior surgical resident at a Chicago area hospital jumped off a tall building after the patient he'd operated on died because he had nicked an artery. I could think of many other similar stories.

The next day, a Saturday, Shorty returned. He remained quiet.

"Sientes algún dolor?" I asked him in my limited Spanish.

He shook his head no, that he wasn't having any pain.

The chairman also happened to be in the clinic, and I asked him to see Shorty.

"At least it's not any worse," he remarked.

On Sunday, I drove to Reedley to check on Shorty.

Shorty, who was single, lived in a spartan, one-room apartment provided by the owner of the farm. Gus lived next door in a cottage with his wife and four children.

With a head-mounted microscope with light, I examined Shorty's eye. The wound remained unchanged.

I lost many nights of sleep, feeling very bad for Shorty and angry with myself for being careless.

I saw him daily for three weeks in a row, driving to Reedley on the weekends. Finally, I saw a thin, transparent film of tissue growing over the cornea and sclera. Under high magnification, I could actually see the red blood cells in the tiny, transparent vessels rushing to the area, trying to heal. I was convinced that the wound looked better.

It was the most beautiful thing I'd ever seen. I could have kissed Shorty. I almost cried with relief when I realized that he wasn't going to lose his eye.

I reduced his visits to twice a week. It took almost three months for the depression to fill in—the longest three months of my life.

Shorty never complained once.

When I saw him a month later, he had a big smile on his face.

"Me siento bien," he said.

He had been back at work. He and Gus had brought us a box of succulent white peaches.

Chapter 13

The Right Place at the Right Time

IT HAD BEEN A BUSY MONDAY. I was in the third year of my eye residency, and we'd just finished with the afternoon clinic. I decided to head over to the radiology department to check on the X-ray films of a patient who'd been admitted Sunday night with a facial fracture involving the orbit. Since VMC didn't have an ENT residency, patients with these fractures were usually managed by the ophthalmology and/or oral surgery (maxillofacial surgery) residents.

Alex Alexander, the third-year resident in oral surgery, had worked closely with me on similar cases. He'd dealt with a lot more facial fractures than I had, but when he had severely injured patients who needed blood gas studies, he often asked me for help. He'd done his training in dental school, without an internship in general surgery, so he often felt inadequate putting a needle deep into someone's groin, into the femoral artery, to get the arterial blood. For critically ill patients, it was important to find out how oxygenated the arterial blood was, as blood from the veins didn't help. Getting arterial blood was difficult because the arteries were deeper in the tissue and couldn't be seen, whereas we could usually see the more superficial veins.

This patient had other injuries too, and Alex needed a blood gas study, so in the middle of the night I'd gone in and done a femoral artery stick, which showed the patient was getting enough oxygen and his life wasn't in any danger.

It was about 4:30 pm in the radiology department. Alex and I were looking at the patient's films to decide what we should do to repair the fracture. It looked like the right orbital floor was fractured into several pieces, and we would probably need to place a sheet of synthetic material like silastic, made of a form of silicone, to create a new orbital floor. This would support the eye and its muscles, keeping them from being trapped in the fracture. If that happened, the eye would be frozen and unable to move.

As we were looking at the films in the viewing room with the radiologist, there was a commotion in the room next door, the interventional radiology procedure room. A woman was undergoing a procedure called an arteriogram—also called an angiogram or angiography.

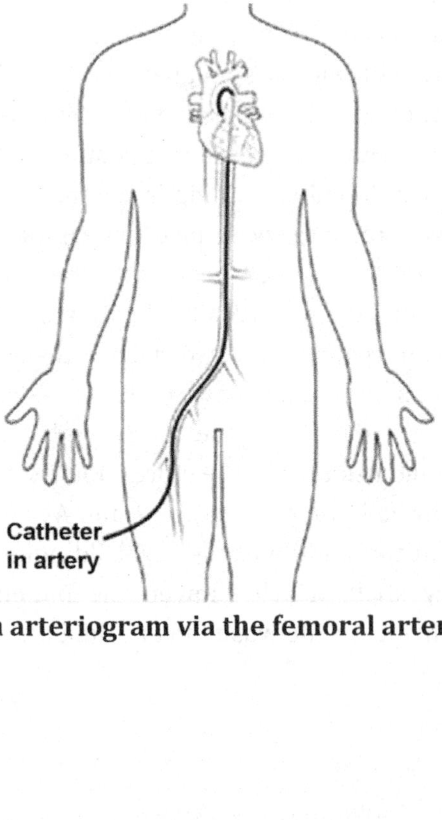

An arteriogram via the femoral artery

This procedure produces an image of the arteries. During the procedure, a thin tube (catheter) is placed in the femoral artery (groin area) through a small nick in the skin, about the size of a pencil tip. The catheter is guided to the area to be studied, and a contrast dye is then injected into the catheter while X-rays are taken. The images will show the dyed blood flowing through the arteries and reveal any blockages.

The woman who was undergoing the angiogram suddenly cried out that her right eye had gone completely dark. She was a woman in her fifties who'd lived with diabetes for many years, and she'd been admitted for evaluation of her coronary arteries following a heart attack.

One of the known risks of such a procedure is that the catheter inside the arteries could dislodge a cholesterol plaque, which may cause a stroke.

The radiologist who'd just injected the dye immediately knew what had happened.

Fortunately, I was in the room next door, and when I heard that the woman couldn't see, I rushed in and asked if I could help.

I happened to be carrying my black bag, as I was planning to make rounds to see my patients after viewing the films. With my ophthalmoscope, I looked into the woman's right eye and noted a classic Central Retinal Artery Occlusion (CRAO).

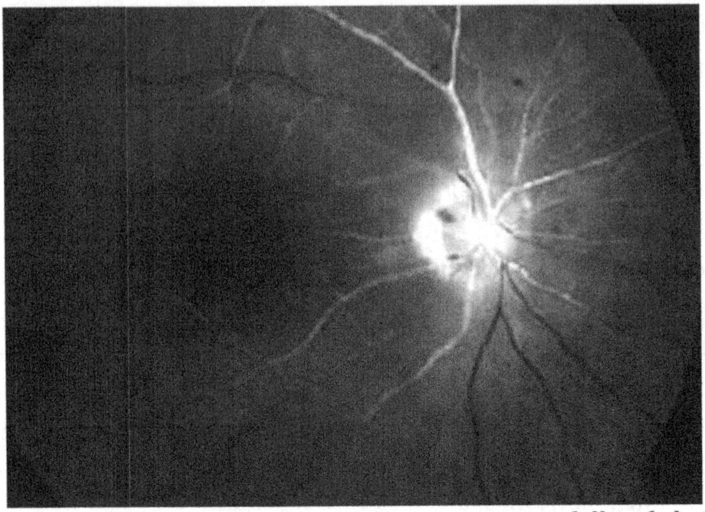

The arterioles inside the right eye were full of bright cholesterol crystals, blocking the circulation, causing ischemia, and slowly killing the retinal tissues as well as the optic nerve.

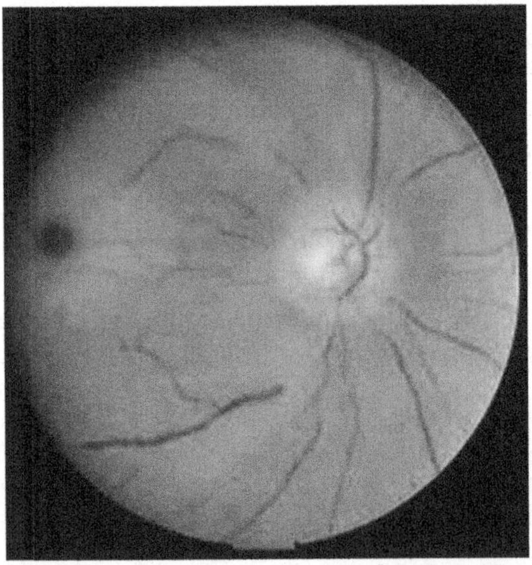

A typical picture of a **Central Retinal Artery Occlusion** showing edema of the optic nerve as well as the macula and parts of the retina.

I'd seen many CRAOs before, but usually they'd happened hours or days before, and by then there was nothing I could do. Patients with sudden visual loss in one eye rarely went to the emergency room acutely; in most cases they would see an optometrist, ophthalmologist or primary care physician and likely be referred to a specialist from there. With the delayed diagnosis, it was too late for effective treatment. If the blockage wasn't cleared within half an hour (some studies suggested an hour at the most), the damage would be permanent. The patient would lose their central vision, resulting in vision of less than 20/200. In some cases, they'd lose even more vision than that.

Although I'd never treated a patient with CRAO in the acute phase, I'd done a great deal of reading about it so I would be prepared if it did happen.

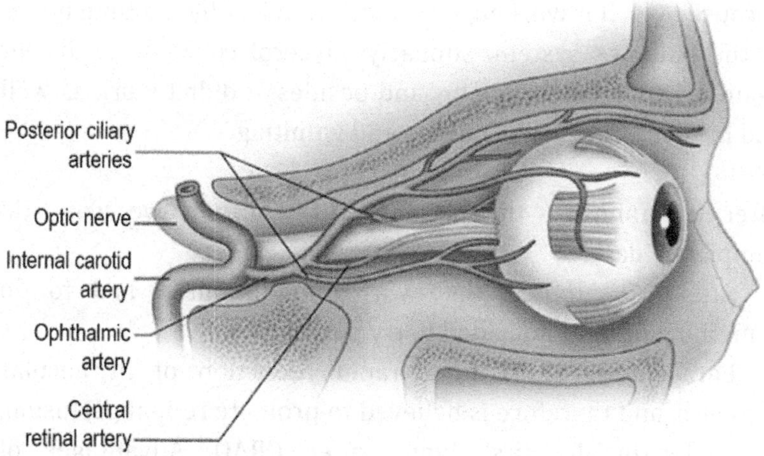

The internal carotid artery is in our neck, which divides into the ophthalmic artery, which nourishes most of the eye, and the central retinal artery (a branch of the ophthalmic artery), which nourishes the optic nerve and macula (i.e., our reading vision).

The radiologist asked me to do what I could. I asked the patient to breathe into a paper bag. This would raise the CO_2

concentration of the air she was breathing, which in turn would send a signal to the vessels to dilate. Sometimes the dilation would cause the cholesterol crystals to move further down, sparing the macula—the part of the eye we read with.

While she was breathing into the paper bag, I applied pressure to the afflicted eye (which we call ocular massage), then released, and repeated the process. I'd read that sometimes the changing pressure inside the eye would dislodge the cholesterol crystal blockage.

While I was massaging her eye, I thought about using Isosorbide to lower the eye pressure, but decided that it wouldn't work because it would take too long.

Isosorbide is an oral hyperosmotic agent, which has been used to reduce intraocular pressure and help dislodge the blockage. But the onset of action wouldn't help in this case, because even if it worked, it would be too late by the time it was in the patient's system. Similarly, glycerol could be used, but again it would take too long, and besides, it didn't work as well and had side effects like nausea and vomiting.

After ten minutes, the patient said that her eye was still completely dark.

After 15 minutes, time was running out. I had to do something drastic. I decided to try paracentesis.

Paracentesis leads to a rapid reduction of intraocular pressure, and therefore is believed to promote retinal perfusion, especially in the first hours after CRAO. Advantages of paracentesis are that the implementation is quick and involves low costs and few resources.

I called up the eye clinic and asked the first-year resident to bring me a new bottle of Proparacaine, some antibiotic drops and a minor surgery tray.

Proparacaine eye drops are used to numb the eye before surgery, certain tests and other procedures. They're designed to prevent pain during the procedures. Proparacaine belongs to the group of medicines called local anesthetics. It works by blocking the pain signals at the nerve endings in the eye.

Every minute counted now, as the retinal tissues were dying without oxygen.

I told the nurse to give the patient 5 mg of Valium in her IV to help sedate her further. I then painted her lids and the surrounding areas with Betadine solution to sterilize the procedure field. With a wire speculum retracting the eyelids, I kept the eye open and instilled a few drops of the anesthetic on her cornea, followed by antibiotic drops to prevent infection when I stuck the needle into her eye.

With a half-inch long 30 gauge needle (one of the smallest gauges) and syringe, and with a gentle thrust at about the 9 o'clock position of the limbus—the area between the transparent cornea and the white sclera—the needle tip entered the anterior chamber, avoiding the iris and the lens. I drew about ½ cc of clear fluid into the syringe, and removed the needle from the eye. The patient didn't feel any pain, just some pressure from my fingers resting on her forehead.

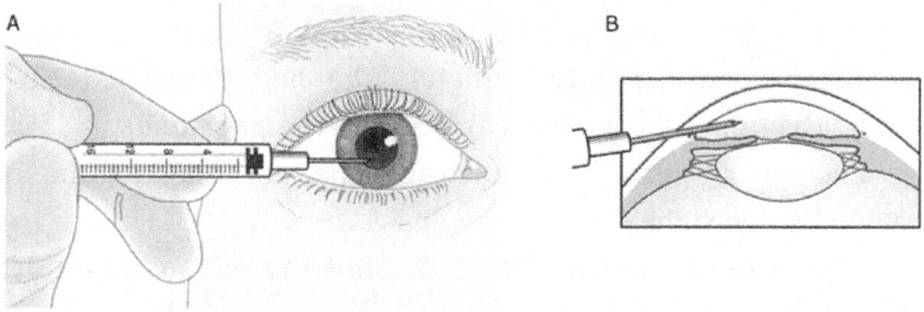

A Paracentesis

A fourth-year medical student from USC who was doing a clerkship in radiology was observing. She began to feel faint as she watched me stick the needle in the woman's eye and had to sit down and put her head between her legs.

Almost immediately the patient exclaimed, "I can see again!" I looked into her eye, and indeed most of the cholesterol crystals had moved further away, and the color of the macula had returned to normal. Her central vision had been restored.

There was a loud cheer from everyone in the room, except for the medical student who was still sitting in the chair, half dazed.

Later, she asked me how I could stick a needle in someone's eye.

"This is medicine," I replied. "You see someone do it, then you read about it, and perhaps practice on a pig eye, and then you do it. I'm sure you'll be able to do it too someday, if you go into ophthalmology. But most non-ophthalmologists simply aren't comfortable with this procedure, because you can do real damage to the eye if you do it incorrectly."

It was one of the rare instances when CRAO was treated in time, simply because an ophthalmologist happened to be nearby and happened to know what to do.

The patient, Mrs. Donna Grey, did have some blockage of her coronary arteries but didn't require bypass surgery. Because of her many decades with diabetes, she had developed early diabetic retinopathy and was followed in the eye clinic.

Each year I got a Christmas card from her, thanking me for saving her eyesight.

The incident happened in 1979, but the memories of Mrs. Grey on the X-ray table still remain fresh in my mind.

There have been major advances in the treatment of strokes since then, such as systemic anticoagulation, systemic venous thrombolysis and catheter-guided intra-arterial fibrinolysis—but none of these are helpful for CRAO, even though it is a form of stroke. It still has to be treated within the crucial time of the first hour, or the damage is irreversible.

Chapter 14

My First Cataract Surgery

THE THREE YEARS OF OPHTHALMOLOGY RESIDENCY was well structured. As mentioned earlier, in the first year we mostly took care of minor problems like infections of the eyes and eyelids or removal of foreign bodies on the cornea, all the while trying to learn how to use the operating microscope and gain as much knowledge about eye diseases as possible.

During the second year, we got to do surgery on the eye muscles to correct strabismus (eyes pointing in different directions), while sometimes watching or assisting in the senior resident's cataract surgeries.

In our senior year, we began to do cataract surgery—a very unforgiving procedure, as the eye is small and the cataract very delicate.

In preparation for the third year, we would try doing surgery on pig eyes, which we got from the slaughterhouse. Using the microscope, I would practice cataract surgery on the pig eye just as if I was doing a real surgery. Of course, the pig eye was quite different from a human eye, but nevertheless it was good preparation for the real surgery, giving us an idea of the steps involved as well as the feel of the tissue when we cut into it.

Toward the end of my second year, I began to look for my first cataract patient. The ideal choice would be someone who was calm, with a high pain and discomfort threshold and large eyes that were easily accessible. Deep-set eyes wouldn't be a good idea because it would be like working in a hole. Someone with tight eyelids and protruding eyes wouldn't be a good idea either because such eyes have a tendency to exert pressure on the eye during surgery. Increased eye pressure during surgery could be very dangerous because it might cause the contents of the eye to extrude through the surgical wound. That would be a catastrophe.

Ruby Connor seemed to be the perfect candidate. She was a quiet, reserved woman in her early seventies who was still working as a bookkeeper for a large packinghouse in the nearby town of Sanger.

In spite of having private insurance and Medicare, Ruby continued to come to VMC because she and her family had been coming since she was a child. She had muscle surgery on her left eye when she was six years old for her wandering eye, i.e., a tendency to turn out. She was very pleased with the surgery, which had been done by an ophthalmologist who was still in town and by then over ninety years old.

Earlier in the year, she came into the clinic because of persistent tearing in her left eye. I explained to her that her tear duct was blocked, and the treatment would be to put silicone tubing through the tear duct, leaving the tube for at least six months, to keep the tear duct open. I advised her that it was a delicate surgery and offered to refer her to another ophthalmologist who specialized in this area, called ocular plastic surgery. But she insisted that I do it. I had assisted in several such procedures, and since it was a procedure on the eyelid, there was little risk of complications involving the sight. So, I decided to do the surgery, which went very well. When I removed the silicone tubing six months later, she no longer had the tearing problem and she was very pleased.

We got along very well and trusted each other. I thought my first cataract patient should be a calm person who trusted me, because if there were any complications, he or she wouldn't go berserk.

Later, Ruby presented as the perfect choice when she began having problems with her bookkeeping work and wanted her cataracts out.

In 1978, cataract surgery began going through some major advances. I was still being taught the traditional way of ICCE, or intra-capsular cataract surgery, which involved removal of the entire lens. The wound was a semicircular incision around the cornea. After removing the entire cataract, the wound would be closed with ten to twelve sutures and the patient would be immobilized in the hospital for a day or two, then recover at home for several weeks.

Since the mid-1980s, this surgery has rarely been done.

When the day for my first cataract surgery arrived, Ruby was ready and I was ready. By then, I was comfortable using the operating microscope. We got set up in the operating room, with me seated behind Ruby's head, and the supervising ophthalmologist sitting next to me.

Under the microscope, all my movements looked greatly exaggerated. I was tense. The supervising attending, Dr. Grayman, an older doctor in his late seventies, was a kind and patient man. I had no awareness that my hand was shaking, but under magnification, there was a tiny tremor that was embarrassingly obvious to my attending and me.

I took a deep breath and steadied myself. I had given Ruby an injection below her right eyeball, a procedure called retro-bulbar anesthesia, to immobilize as well as numb the eye.

With a pair of forceps in my left hand and micro scissors in my right, I made an incision at the nine o'clock position in the conjunctiva and extended it to the three o'clock position. With a sharp blade, I made a stab at the limbus (the area between the cornea and sclera), and I entered the anterior chamber of the eye at the twelve o'clock position, extending the incision to the right and then left.

Ruby shifted a little, and in the microscope it was like watching an earthquake. I calmly said, "Ruby, things are going well. Just try to keep still."

Once the anterior chamber was opened, I irrigated a solution called alpha-chymotrypsin (an enzyme) to dissolve the lens zonules so that the lens could be removed more easily.

I gingerly placed the cryo probe tip on the anterior surface of the lens, and stepped on the pedal of the cryo machine. Soon an ice ball formed and extended to the entire lens. I gently rocked back and forth a little, then withdrew the probe along with the frozen lens at the tip. The entire lens that had turned cloudy was safely removed from Ruby's eye.

Carefully, I picked up the IOL (intraocular lens) with special micro-forceps, and placed it just in front of the iris.

"It looks centered, Jim," Dr. Grayman remarked.

I examined the position of the IOL carefully and noted that it was indeed centered. This was an old-fashioned anterior chamber IOL that we placed in front of the iris, in contrast to the IOLs now that are placed behind the iris.

Immediately and gingerly, I placed a 10-0 nylon suture at the twelve o'clock position, and then added a suture on each side. In eye surgery, we try not to leave the eye wound open because if the patient should cough or move, it might cause pressure to build up and the contents in the eye to extrude through the wound.

I gently tapped the eyeball and noted that the IOL didn't move. Feeling confident that the IOL was in the correct position, I placed the rest of the sutures. I then buried the knots of the suture under the sclera to prevent irritation under the eyelids. The conjunctiva was then pulled down to drape over the sclera and the sutures.

I leaned back and let out a sigh of relief.

"Good job," said Dr. Grayman.

"Ruby, we're finished," I announced. "Thanks for being such a good patient."

The nurse helped Ruby onto a gurney and wheeled her to the recovery room.

As soon as Ruby was out of the room, I jumped up the air with joy and did a little dance. I'd done my first cataract with IOL and it went perfectly well!

Dr. Grayman smiled and threw up his hand to give me a high five.

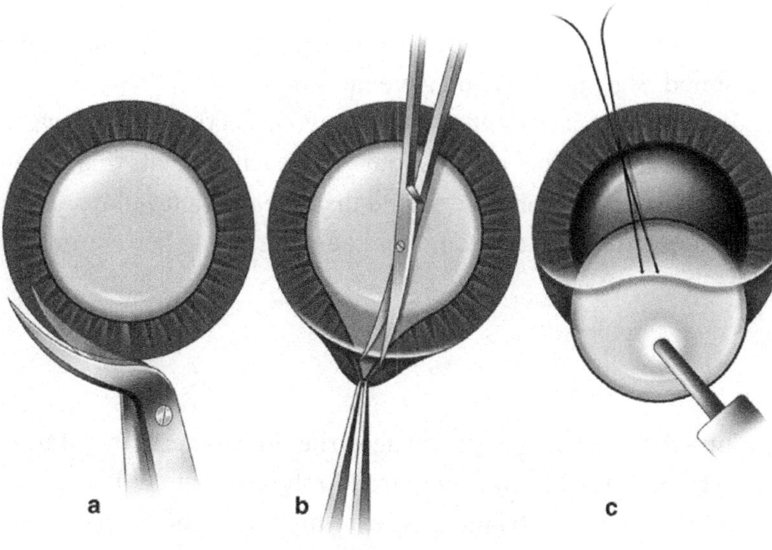

Intra-capsular cataract extraction
a: Incision with curved scissors.
b: Peripheral iridectomy
c: Cryo probe to remove the cataract

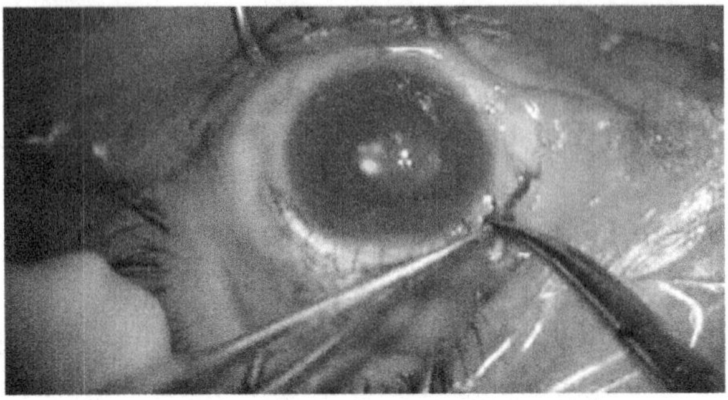

Intra-capsular cataract extraction with anterior chamber IOL

The next morning, Ruby came into the clinic with a big smile on her face.

"Dr. Hung, I had forgotten how bright the colors are," she exclaimed. She stood up and gave me a hug.

Her vision was 20/40 without any correction. There was a little edema on her cornea, but I'd learned that this often happened post-surgery and would disappear in a few days.

"I hope you can do your bookkeeping work better now," I said.

***

Looking back over 45 years ago, the intra-capsular cataract extraction seemed brutal compared to the current methods.

While I was in training, great improvements were being made in cataract surgery as well as in IOL technology. It seemed that I was constantly learning new things.

During the latter part of my third year in training, I learned ECCE—extra-capsular cataract surgery—and then shortly after I went into private practice, I had to learn the phacoemulsification technique.

Now, the intra-capsular cataract extraction that I did on Ruby is rarely done and the anterior chamber IOL rarely used. Most cataract surgeries are now done with phacoemulsification.

Also known as "phaco," it's the most common technique used for cataract removal nowadays. Usually, it takes no more than half an hour to remove a cataract through phacoemulsification, and that too requiring only minimal sedation, i.e., local anesthesia (injecting anesthesia around the eye) or topical anesthesia (administering numbing drops into the eye).

This cataract procedure requires a small surgical incision around the edge of the cornea, creating an opening through the membrane surrounding the lens. The next step involves inserting a small ultrasonic probe into the opening to break up the cloudy lens into tiny fragments using sound waves, which act as a microscopic jackhammer. An attachment on the probe tip is then used for suction of broken-down cataract fragments.

Once the lens particles are removed, an intraocular lens implant is placed inside the natural lens capsule. A hollowed-out tube is used by the ophthalmologists to insert the IOL through a tiny corneal incision.

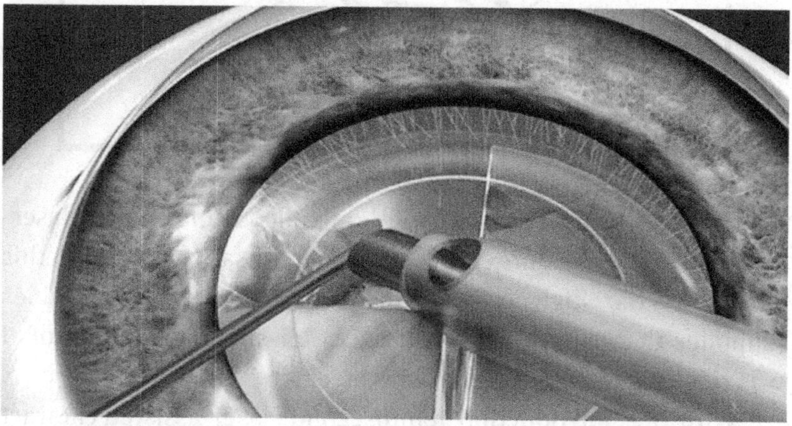

Phacoemulsification, removing the cataract with ultrasound

Extra-capsular cataract surgery
Nowadays, this cataract procedure is used in cases of highly advanced cataracts that are too dense for phacoemulsification, or when phacoemulsification isn't possible for various other reasons.

A slightly larger incision is required for this technique, so that the cataract can be removed in one piece instead of being fragmented within the eye. Just like phacoemulsification, an artificial lens (IOL) is placed inside the same capsular bag.

A number of sutures are required to close the comparatively larger wound, which also results in slower recovery of the wound as well as visual function.

In developing countries, ECCE has greatly improved, and now can be done through a small incision that doesn't even require any sutures to close the wound. It has proven to be as safe and effective as phacoemulsification.

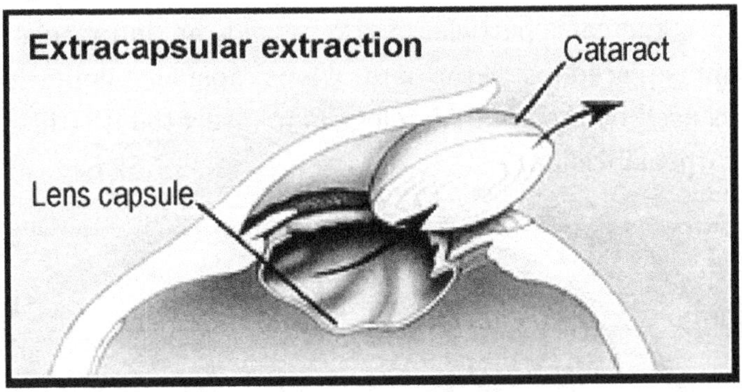

Now there's an even newer method called femtosecond laser-assisted cataract surgery. The major disadvantage of this surgery is the high cost of the laser and the disposables (supplies that can only be used once) for surgery. In addition, I was told that the learning curve is steep.

With its introduction, femtosecond laser-assisted cataract surgery was believed to have revolutionized cataract surgery.

However, the judgment of clinical benefit was found to be far more complex than initially thought and the benefits few, compared to phacoemulsification. The results of the surgery don't seem to be any better than phaco, just much more expensive.

Femtosecond laser-assisted cataract surgery is out of question for developing countries because of the prohibitively expensive laser and the disposable supplies needed for each case. There's no way any developing country can even afford phacoemulsification, let alone femtosecond laser assisted cataract surgery, when small incision extra-capsular cataract surgery costs pretty much nothing aside from the cost of the IOL.

Recalling the day I did my first cataract surgery so many years ago, I still relive the excitement and pride of accomplishment I felt to have learned how to do this very delicate and sight-saving procedure.

Chapter 15
Bishop

During my ophthalmology residency, I did quite a bit of moonlighting working in the ER. I had signed up with a company in San Francisco that had contracts with hospitals all over California, providing them with ER coverage.

At the time, I thought it was such big money—$20 to $30 an hour—especially compared to not many years ago in college when I was making $1.25 to $1.75 an hour. I guess everything in life is relative. At that point, I really had no idea how much ophthalmologists made. Later, when I went into private practice as a retina surgeon, I was surprised to be paid several hundred dollars for a laser treatment, something that took less than half an hour. I thought perhaps I had wasted my life working so many weekends in the ER.

But what is life but a summation of one's experiences? The more experiences one has, the richer one's life is. Looking back over forty-five years ago, I'm glad that I worked in those ERs. My life is so much richer because of those experiences.

The hospital I normally worked in was the Visalia Community Hospital, in Visalia, a town about an hour's drive south of Fresno. But one day, I got a call from the secretary of the company in San Francisco saying that they would like me to work in Bishop. I had no idea where Bishop was. I was told that they would pay for my airfare and the rate would be $30/hour.

Having always been adventurous, I thought it would be a new experience, and since I'd worked for almost a year in the Natividad Medical Center as chief resident, taking care of all sorts of seriously ill patients, I was confident that I could handle almost anything that arrived at the ER.

Later, Mary and I went over to visit our next door neighbors, Elmer and Nettie, an older couple who'd been very kind to us, and with whom we'd become good friends. They were especially fond of our daughter, Melissa, now almost three years old. I told them that I would be working in Bishop.

"Bishop!" exclaimed Elmer. "Jim, that's the most dangerous airport. There have been so many crashes up there." Elmer had worked in Bishop as the foreman for a major construction company and knew the area well.

"Oh no, what I have done?" I exclaimed. "Perhaps I can tell the company I've changed my mind. Is it possible for me to drive there?"

Elmer shook his head. "When you look at the map, it doesn't look like Bishop is that far away from Fresno, but there's no direct road, because from here to Bishop is mostly mountain. To drive there, you'd have to drive south almost to LA, and then drive north. It would take you the entire day to get there," he commented.

The next day, I called the company and indicated that I'd changed my mind and couldn't work in Bishop. The secretary explained that they'd tried contacting many doctors on their employment register, but none of them were available and now it was too late to find another doctor. It looked like I was headed for Bishop after all.

It was a weekend assignment. I would work from 5 pm on a Friday to Sunday afternoon, and I would catch a 5:30 flight back to Fresno. For that, I would be paid $1,440. It was too good to pass up.

Friday afternoon, Mary drove me to the Fresno Air Terminal. The plane was a 4-seater. I sat next to the pilot and there were two other passengers. The flight was bumpy but not jarring, and the pilot, a man in his fifties, was reassuring.

"I know, some of you have heard how dangerous the Bishop airport is," he remarked. "I've been flying from Bishop to all over California for over thirty years, and I've never had any mishaps." I felt better.

I learned later from the ER nurse that because of the high altitude and mountains, the winds could change direction without warning. Usually it was the unpredictable strong winds that caused problems for the less experienced pilots.

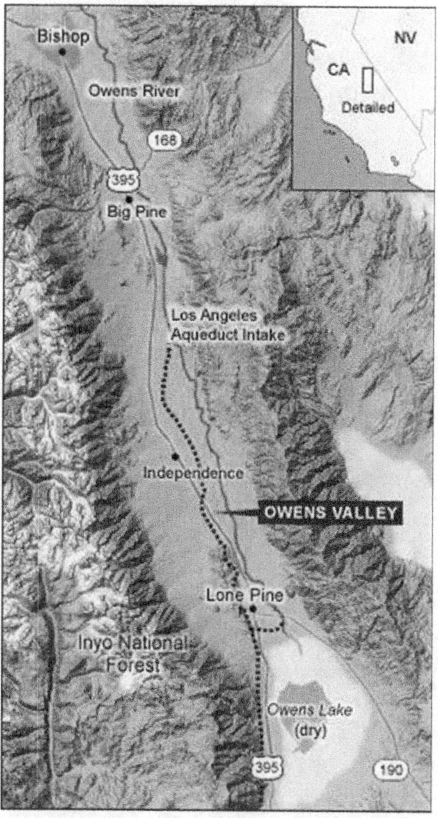

Bishop, high in the mountains

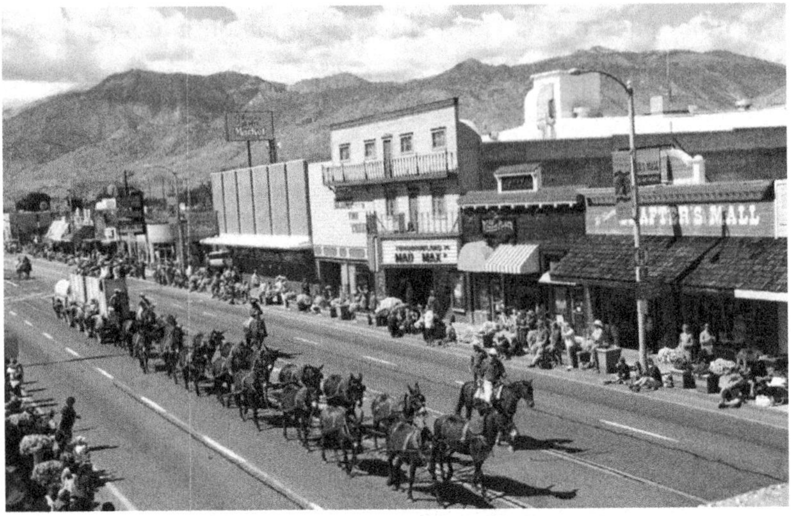

Mule Day Parade in Bishop

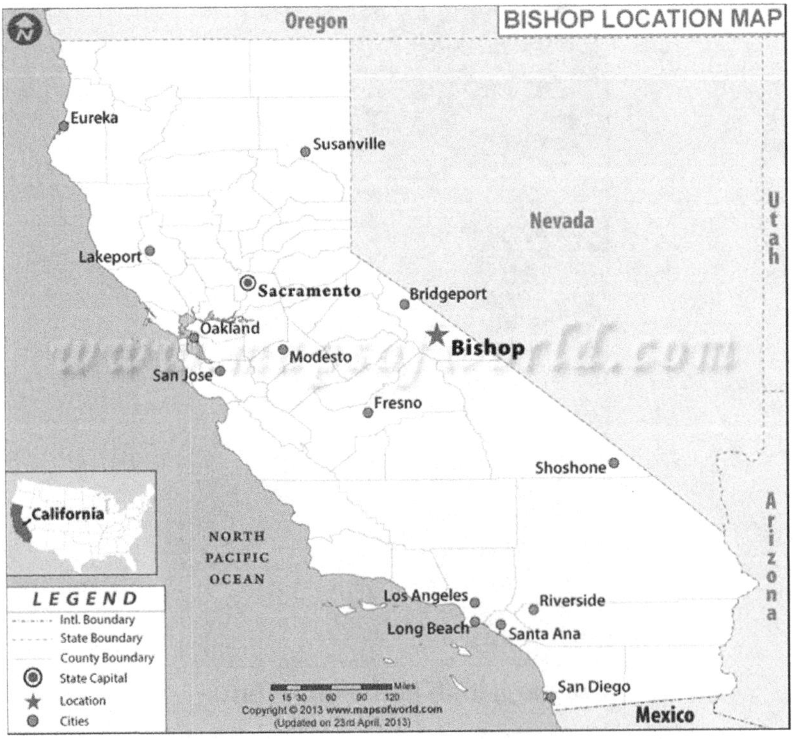

Bishop in relation to the rest of California

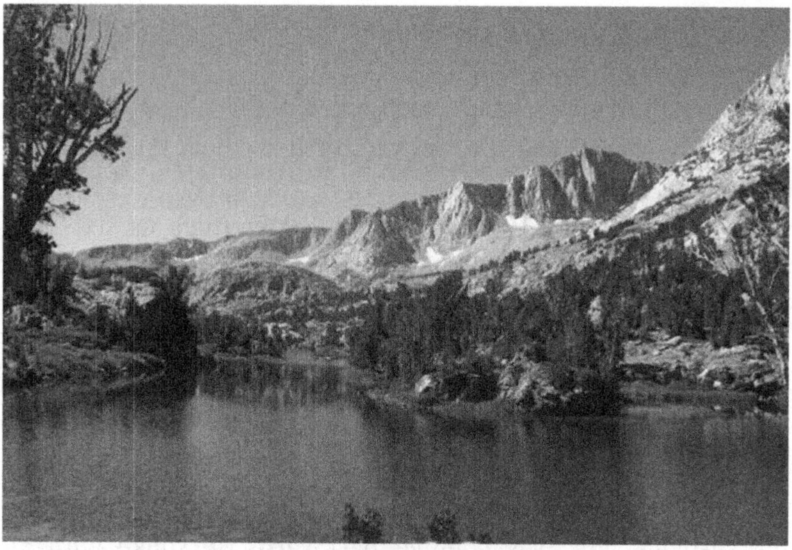

Scenery around Bishop

The head ER nurse picked me up at the small Bishop airport. Nancy was a woman of about fifty with an athletic build, short blond hair and large blue eyes. She reminded me of Doris Day. She was starting her shift at 5 pm as well. On the way to the hospital, she gave me a rundown of the kinds of patients they usually saw in the ER.

It was now September, and most of the summer tourists had left the area, so hopefully the weekend at the hospital wouldn't be too busy.

In addition to my responsibilities in the ER, I was also responsible for all the inpatients so the doctors in town didn't have to be on call constantly.

When we arrived, the doctor who was leaving signed out to me and told me that there was only one patient he was worried about.

It was their only patient in the ICU: a man in his early sixties who'd had a massive stroke. He was on the ventilator and his vital signs were unstable. The other doctor suggested that I keep a close eye on him, and then headed off to catch his flight to San Francisco via Fresno.

I was shown my room, which was a regular hospital room. I put on my white jacket and went directly to the ICU to check on the patient on ventilator.

Mr. Ward, a big man who looked older than his sixty-odd years of age, had his eyes closed. Next to him was Larry, the respiratory therapist, who was suctioning the tube in Mr. Ward's trachea.

Larry was a tall, strong man over six feet tall in his mid-forties who had retired from the Army a few years ago and decided to have a second career as a respiratory therapist. His square face and prominent chin had been scarred by acne and his jet-black hair was combed backward. He spoke with an accent that sounded like those I'd heard in cowboy movies.

"Doc, good to see you," Larry drawled, extending his right hand to shake mine.

"How is Mr. Ward doing?" I asked.

"He's been fighting the tube," Larry responded. "I think maybe he's ready to have it out."

"When was his last blood gas?" I asked.

"I don't know. I think it was a few days ago," he replied.

As I'd been working in ERs for a few years, I was familiar with what I should and shouldn't do. My chief responsibility was to take care of all patients coming to the ER, and to take care of the inpatients only if they had new problems. As all the inpatients had their own doctors, it wasn't my job to make any treatment decisions unless it was something urgent or an emergency that couldn't wait until their regular doctors saw them on Monday. I was there to cover the hospital patients so the local doctors, especially the primary care docs, could have a break. I knew these primary care docs worked very hard, and they didn't need to be awakened at night or come in over the weekends for all sorts of minor problems that could be handled by someone like me.

I thought it was inappropriate for Larry to suggest that Mr. Ward might be ready to have his tube out. The decision wasn't his or mine—it should be made by Mr. Ward's regular doctor. It struck me as a red flag. After working in hospitals for years, I realized that sometimes people had hidden agendas, and they weren't always what was best for the patients.

I went over Mr. Ward's charts, and noted that his blood pressure hadn't been stable and he was on several medications to control it.

At dinnertime, Nancy joined me.

"Doctor Hung, I think you should be aware of Larry," she whispered.

Surprised, I asked, "Why?"

"He's always trying to talk the new docs into doing things that would make his life easier," she replied. "Mr. Ward is a lot of work for him because he has to keep his tubing clean by suction, and also, because Mr. Ward has been fighting the tube, Larry has to adjust it. He just doesn't want to do the work," she finished with a shake of her head.

I learned early on in medical school to always listen to the nurses, because some of them had been around for a long time and knew how to deal with most situations.

"Thanks for the tip," I said. "It's important for me to know."

It was very busy in the ER that evening. We saw a twelve-year-old girl with severe asthma, and the inhalers weren't working for her. I started an IV to hydrate her, which usually helped in such attacks, and gave her several kinds of drugs to help her breathe, as well as prednisone to reduce inflammation. In addition, I ordered a breathing treatment for her by Larry that involved medications being sprayed into her lungs.

After two hours at the ER, the girl's wheezing had stopped and she was feeling much better. She was discharged soon after.

Another patient was a ten-year-old boy who was hit above his right upper eyelid by a pebble from a slingshot and had a laceration, which I closed with several sutures.

Later on, a middle-aged woman arrived with a severe headache. Nancy told me that she was a regular and usually a shot of Demerol took care of the problem. I had encountered many patients with headaches before and I was very conservative about giving out narcotics. But in this case, since the nurse knew the patient, I wasn't ready to do a long workup on her, since she had a regular doctor who could follow up with her.

Before I retired to my room, I decided to visit each patient again to see if anyone needed sleeping medication, so I could do it before going to bed rather than being awakened later.

In the ICU, Larry was again suctioning the tube in Mr. Ward's trachea.

"Doc, he's really bucking the tube," said Larry. "I think he is ready to be ex-tubated."

"Larry, this is a tough decision and I usually let the attending doc make it," I replied. "I'd hate to take it out only to find that we have to put it back in. It would be a disaster. Especially for a combative patient like that—it would be very difficult to put the tube back in without an anesthesiologist."

Larry looked disappointed.

"Since he's fighting the tube, I can give him a little Valium to relax his muscles. Maybe that would stop the bucking," I remarked.

The ICU nurse standing next to us said, "That's a good idea."

"How about 5 mg of Valium IV?" I asked.

The nurse promptly got a vial of Valium and injected it into Mr. Ward's IV. Soon, he stopped fighting the tube and became more restful.

To my surprise, I went to bed at midnight and woke up at 6, with six straight hours of sleep. I marveled at what a good deal this was, being paid $30 an hour for sleeping on the job!

As I was having breakfast, I was paged to the ER.

A twenty-year-old college student had been hiking with her boyfriend when she was bitten on her left ankle by a rattlesnake. She said she was certain it was a rattlesnake.

The day ER nurse, Betty, knew exactly what to do. She got out the anti-venom, and with my approval, injected the student.

Betty remarked, "Doctor Hung, we take care of bites like this almost monthly during the summer time. We know exactly what kind of snakes are in the area."

Soon, the college student, Dolores, was sitting up in the gurney, with her left foot elevated. She was admitted for observation.

Betty told me that she had treated many snakebites in Bishop, and had never encountered anyone who had died from it. I took it as a good sign—I certainly didn't want any patients to die on my watch.

As Dolores was being admitted, a young man arrived with a bloody face. He had fallen from his mountain bike, and his face met the ground. He broke two front teeth and suffered a large laceration on the chin.

Betty cleaned off the wound, and I injected the area with 2% Lidocaine. The wound was closed with a number of nylon sutures.

I put the two broken teeth in saline.

"I don't know if the dentist can put them back," I said to the young man. "They look jagged. I can contact the dentist on call to see if anything can be done."

"Oh, my dad's a dentist in town," the young man replied. "I'll give him a call."

He went to make the phone call, and I was later told that his father didn't think the two teeth could be put back in.

I made my rounds on all the patients, and answered the nurses' questions. Sometimes they weren't sure about orders the attending doctors had written, such as the dosage and frequency, and I had to write new orders in some cases

It seemed pretty quiet in the hospital except for Mr. Ward, who was again fighting his tube. I told the nurse to repeat the Valium every three hours if he remained agitated.

At lunchtime, Larry again tried to talk me into having Mr. Ward's tube removed.

I was getting a little irritated and said, "Larry, my job here is to take care of urgent needs and emergencies. Mr. Ward's situation is neither. I don't want to do something that isn't good for the patient, or something that would make his doctor mad at me. It's not my job to have the tube removed. It's up to his doctor.

"To be honest with you," I continued, "I've never intubated a moving patient. I really wouldn't know what to do if I had to put the tube back in and he started fighting me. I'm not going to rock the boat while I'm here just for the weekend. I don't want anyone to die on my watch."

"Doc, I'm sorry if you think I'm trying to push you to take his tube out," Larry remarked in an almost inaudible voice.

Betty, who was sitting across the table, smiled and winked at me, as if to say I was right to tell Larry off.

Later that day, I stopped by the snakebite patient's room. Dolores' left leg had been elevated and the swelling hadn't increased. She was comfortable with the IV morphine drip, as I'd been told snakebites could be very painful.

She was watching *All in the Family* on TV, a sitcom I often watched on Saturday evenings at home. I decided to sit down, watching and laughing with her and her mother.

After dinner, I stopped by the ER desk. Nancy was on shift now, drinking a cup of coffee. As she handed me a cup as well, I asked, "Nancy, how long have you lived in Bishop?"

"Doc, I was born here," she answered. "My family is one of the original families that founded this town. My great-great-grandfather came to California with Mr. Bishop to explore this area."

"I've lived in Fresno for years, and I had no idea that Bishop was so close," I remarked.

"It's usually a quiet place. It's in a large county with few people. Bishop is the largest town in Inyo County and there are less than 4,000 residents in the city, and perhaps another 10,000 in the greater Bishop area," Nancy explained.

"How do you like living here?" I asked.

"I really like it up here," she replied. "It's a safe and quiet place. There's almost no crime except during tourist season when outsiders come and commit petty crimes. There's so much to do here for recreation. The Mammoth Mountain Sky Resort is less than an hour's drive away. There's good fishing in the river, and so many hiking trails.

"The landscape near Bishop is some of the best natural scenery in California, so we get a lot of wildlife photographers. People come here for hunting, rock climbing, hiking and fishing.

"One thing I feel bad about in this area is its history," she added.

"Why?" I asked.

"It's how the native people were treated," she said.

"You mean there were Indians here?" I asked.

Nancy nodded. "My grandpa used to tell me stories about this area. Prior to the arrival of Europeans and Americans, the Bishop area was home to a subset of Northern Paiute First Nation. These 'Native American' people were also referred to as Owens Valley Paiute, and before that they were called the Eastern Mono."

"You mean the same Mono tribes as those near Fresno," I interrupted.

"Yes, they were related and spoke the same language," Nancy confirmed. "They were really good hunters and used methods like stalking deer while wearing camouflage, surrounding the deer with people, using trained dogs and sometimes setting brush on fire. Antelope and mountain sheep were caught by driving them into a corral or between rows of rock piles and narrow canyons.

"Interestingly, I learned that they never bothered the bears because they considered them to closely resemble human beings."

Nancy took a sip of her coffee and continued. "In 1846, four years before California gained admission into the Union, more and more people arrived in the area because of Bishop's proximity to the Eastern Sierra Mountain Range, which had a lot of minerals. They attracted miners and prospectors from all over.

"Sadly, these new people gradually squeezed out the natives and destroyed their hunting grounds by raising cattle on the land. In retaliation, Paiute began killing cattle.

"Then a war broke out between the natives and the US Army, volunteers and local settlers in 1862. The natives lost and they were forced to relocate to Fort Tejon a year later," she finished.

"It's a familiar story with the native Indians isn't it?" I commented.

"Sadly, it is," lamented Nancy.

So far, I'd been in Bishop for just over 24 hours, and I was already doing and learning so much.

At that point, a mother brought in her eight-year-old son with an ice pack on his right forearm.

"I think Hank broke his arm," announced his mother. "He was skateboarding and fell."

Hank was a cooperative boy. I examined his arm and noted some swelling, but no misalignment of his arm.

"Let's take some X-rays," I said.

Nancy paged the X-ray technician to come in, and before long the films were available. They revealed a non-displaced fracture of the ulna bone. Hank needed a cast.

I'd put on many casts before and this would be an easy one. I made a cast from Hank's elbow to his wrist, and when it was dry, I drew a smiling face on it with a blue Sharpie pen.

Nancy went over the instructions with Hank's mother about keeping the cast dry, and said that she should call on Monday for an appointment with the orthopedic surgeon to check on the cast.

By that time, it was after 10 pm. I made my rounds on every patient. I checked on Mr. Ward. With the small dose of Valium every three hours as needed, he had since quieted down and was no longer fighting the ventilator.

I retired to my room just before midnight, and again slept until 6 am. I was really lucky to be able to get two full nights of sleep.

After breakfast, I made my rounds again.

Dolores, the young woman with the snakebite, was eating her breakfast when I reached her room. The swelling in her leg had decreased substantially. The area around the bite showed signs of necrosis, i.e., dead tissue that was deep blue, but it was no worse than when she was initially seen. There was no sign of infection.

"I think you can go home today if promise me that you'll keep that leg elevated," I said.

She smiled and nodded.

I wrote orders for her discharge, including instructions to see her family doctor on Monday for follow-up.

Next, I stopped by the ICU. Mr. Ward was still not responsive to verbal commands, but when I pricked him lightly with my safety pin, he withdrew his leg swiftly, meaning that if we'd removed his tube only to find that he still needed it, he would've fought anyone trying to put a tube into his throat.

Larry was nowhere in sight. Perhaps he was embarrassed that I'd called him out on it.

Later, I thought perhaps I shouldn't have been so direct with Larry. I've always hated confrontations; but this one I did without thinking. The words simply came out of my mouth, almost like a reflex.

The rest of the day was uneventful. At 4:30 pm, my replacement came in and I checked out to him, telling him what had transpired with Mr. Ward.

He smiled and said, "That sounds like Larry."

Nancy drove me to the airport and I flew back to Fresno. Despite Elmer's warnings and my own initial concerns, I was very pleased that I'd gone to Bishop.

Chapter 16
Back from the Dead

IN DECEMBER 1978, I was again working in the ER at Visalia Community Hospital. I would usually work from 5 pm on a Friday to 7 am, Monday, which added up to 60 hours. At $25 an hour, I was able to make $1,500 over a weekend. In the 1970s, that was a tremendous amount of money.

As I'd been working there for over two years, I'd gotten to know the people fairly well. Familiar patients would show up week after week—a few with uncontrolled asthma who would come in for breathing treatments, IV fluid and medications; or the usual patients with headaches who asked for and sometimes demanded narcotics. These patients were the most difficult to deal with, because some of them would get belligerent if they were denied narcotics. I'd learned to deal with them by being firm and not giving in. Then there were the usual minor lacerations in children that were easily sutured.

That weekend, I also had a truck driver come in with severe and painful hemorrhoids, which I had to incise to release the pressure.

But one patient worried me. She was a woman in her late forties, very frail with a face as pale as milk. She looked ill and uncomfortable. She'd been in and out of the ER for years because of her heart. She had been under the care of the newly hired hospital cardiologist, Dr. Julia Ong, a woman in her thirties of Chinese heritage, whose parents came from the Philippines and had settled in New Jersey.

Dr. Ong was in New Jersey visiting her parents, and while she was away the ER was responsible for this woman's care.

Martha had been diagnosed with cardiac arrhythmia and Dr. Ong was considering putting in a pacemaker. Everyone at the ER knew Martha well.

I was comfortable with most patients, but I was wary of Martha's condition because I knew how unpredictable issues like hers could be. I'd heard about patients who visited their cardiologist and were given a clean bill of health, only to die of a massive heart attack that night or the next day. Such stories were too familiar and it was weighing on my mind.

On Sunday morning, Martha was brought in again by her husband Roy, a retired army captain. He was a muscular man and a man of authority. Martha was at the ER because of a strange feeling that her heart was beating irregularly and it seemed to flutter. She had no pain or shortness of breath.

Reading EKGs was not my strong area; but there was a consultant service we could fax the tracing to in San Francisco. The consultant's reading was that Martha had cardiac arrhythmia, which we already knew. His recommendation was a pacemaker, which we also already knew Dr. Ong was considering.

In the meantime, what was I to do? Her condition had essentially remained the same since her last visit to the ER, which was just two days ago. Should I admit her to the hospital? But what else could I do for her in the hospital except hook her up to a monitor?

I showed Martha and Roy the interpretation by the consultant cardiologist, and they agreed that there was nothing we could do for her in the hospital at the moment. What she needed was a pacemaker, which they could discuss with Dr. Ong when she returned.

I went over all ten medications Martha was on with her and Roy. There was nothing I could add or thought she should discontinue.

The rest of Sunday was uneventful, with the usual sort of patients reporting coughs, colds, aches and pains.

At midnight, I retired to my bedroom and quickly fell asleep. At 3 am, the nurse woke me to say that Martha was back at the ER She was feeling really odd and her heart was acting strangely.

I again listened to her heart carefully, which produced the familiar sound of arrhythmia that I'd heard before.

Again, I did an EKG and had the tracing sent to San Francisco for interpretation. Again, the consultant cardiologist returned the same answer and said that she needed a pacemaker.

What was I to do?

I'd learned from past experience that if there was any doubt, I should admit the patient, because if anything bad happened I would be covered. But Martha had been in and out of the hospital so many times, and Dr. Ong would be back in the office at 9 am. I thought it would be alright for her to wait until she could see Dr. Ong, which was only a few hours away, so I sent her home.

By now, it was 5:30 am. I went back to sleep and got up at 6:30, ready to drive back to Fresno to begin another day in my last year of ophthalmology residency.

My replacement, Dr. Cohen, had driven in from San Francisco and arrived at the hospital just before 7 am. I was signing out to him and told him about Martha.

As we were drinking our coffee and going over the patients, there was a commotion at the ER entrance. Martha's husband ran in, carrying her on his back.

"Help! Martha's heart had stopped!" Roy yelled.

Dr. Cohen and I rushed to help him, taking Martha off his back and placing her on a gurney. She was completely limp and lifeless. Her face was colorless. She had no pulse and no blood pressure.

Dr. Cohen immediately began CPR and I was able to start an IV in her forearm. She was quickly hooked up to a cardiac monitor, which showed asystole—a flat line.

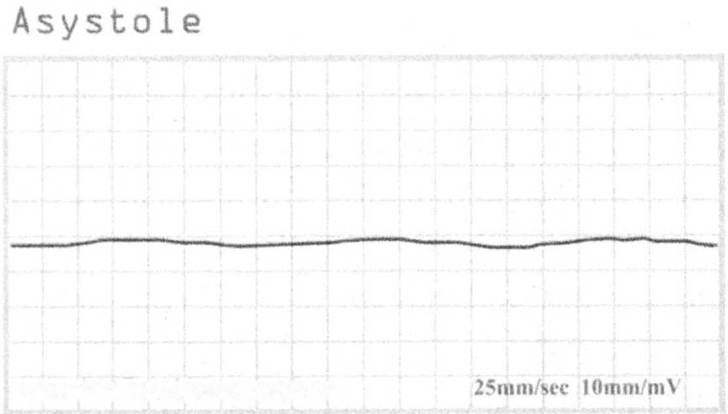

Asystole, colloquially referred to as "flatlining," indicates the cessation of electrical and mechanical heart activity. It's treated with CPR and an intravenous vasopressor like epinephrine (a.k.a. adrenaline).

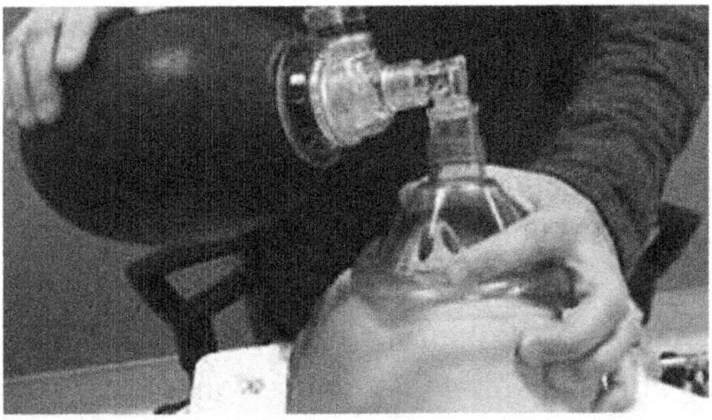

A bag valve mask (BVM), sometimes referred to as an Ambu bag, is a handheld tool that is used to deliver positive pressure ventilation to any subject with insufficient or ineffective breaths. It consists of a self-inflating bag, one-way valve, mask, and an oxygen reservoir.

The respiratory therapist was paged, and he quickly arrived with an Ambu bag and began delivering oxygen into Martha's lungs.

Dr. Cohen continued compressing Martha's heart. Within five minutes, I felt a pulse, indicating that her heart had resumed beating. A short time later, her eyes opened. She seemed confused.

"What happened?" she asked.

"Your heart stopped for a short time," replied Dr. Cohen.

Martha was admitted to the ICU, and I went to talk to her husband.

"What happened?" I asked Roy.

"We were having breakfast, and she just slumped over," Roy explained. "It's a good thing we only live a block away. I carried her to the car and drove here as fast as I could."

"Thanks to your fast action, you saved your wife's life," I said.

Martha was hooked up to a cardiac monitor, and Dr. Ong would be in to see her soon, when she would most likely make the decision to put a pacemaker in.

Before I left, I stopped by Martha's bed and told her that I was so glad her husband had the presence of mind to bring her back to the ER as quickly as he did, and that he'd saved her life.

Martha seemed tired, but she gave me a faint smile.

As I drove to VMC to begin another day of residency, I was shaking my head at what a close call it was. It could have ended very differently, which would've affected so many people's lives.

After the incident, I again reminded myself that if there was ever any question, always admit the patient to the hospital. If Martha had died in hospital, there probably wouldn't be any questions; but if she'd died at home, especially hours after seeing a doctor in the ER, there would be a lot of questions.

The truth of the matter was that it was often impossible to predict how a person's heart was going to behave. I'd read about famous people who died shortly after being reassured by their cardiologist that their heart was fine.

I was so grateful that Roy acted the way he did. I would have felt really bad if she had died.

Martha was one of the few patients who did well after CPR. She had a pacemaker put in the following day.

Having worked in the ER for several years, performing Advanced Cardiac Life Support (ACLS) had become second nature to me. I could be awakened in the middle of the night from a deep sleep, and immediately be able to perform the procedure. I would know exactly the sequence of medications to give the patient. It's one part of being a physician of which I am very proud. I've always regarded myself as a physician first and an ophthalmologist second.

Even though ACLS has been questioned recently as an effective method because of its low success rates, Martha was the kind of patient who should do well because her issue was arrhythmia and all she needed was the pacemaker.

Attempts to resuscitate patients have changed dramatically throughout history, with each new version developed in the hope of saving lives. People have been trying to revive victims whose hearts have stopped for hundreds of years.

One of the early methods was the Flagellation Method, in which rescuers whipped the victim with stinging nettles or struck them with their hands or a wet cloth to stimulate a response.

Another treatment was the Heat Method. Warm ashes, hot water, burning dried animal dung—anything hot—was applied to the abdomen of the victim, which was thought to restore heat and life to a cold body.

In 1530, the Bellows Method was developed. Fireplace bellows were first used by the Swiss physician Paracelsus to introduce air into a patient's lungs. Variations of this method were used in Europe for 300 years.

In 1770, the Inversion Method was used. Lowering the body expelled air from the lungs, and inspiration resulted from lifting the victim. This was used in England, Europe and America with success in drowning cases.

In 1773, the Barrel Method became popular, in which a barrel was rolled back and forth across a victim's chest. The barrel movement backward caused compression of the chest for expiration. Barrel movement forward released the pressure for inspiration.

There were a number of other methods used from 1773 to 1932, at which time the Holger Nielson Method was invented. This method involved lifting the victim's arm upward and pushing down on the victim's back. Until the 1950s, the accepted method of resuscitation was the chest-pressure and arm-lift technique. The method was eventually shown to be ineffective.

In 1958, mouth-to-mouth resuscitation was invented. The rescuer blows into the victim's mouth, keeping the head back and the nose pinched.

In 1960, Cardiopulmonary Resuscitation was standardized, involving the combination of chest compressions and mouth-to-mouth resuscitation. All medical personnel were trained in this method.

Being on the front line of medicine isn't easy. There's so much to know, and unfortunately, the human body often behaves differently and unpredictably.

Working in the ER, I was always worried that a patient would die because of my ignorance, incompetence, not knowing how to do certain procedures or simply bad luck.

As I was writing this story, I learned that a surgeon in Austria recently amputated the wrong leg, i.e., the good leg, much like the story of the incorrect eye being removed. It's a physician's worst nightmare. In my medical career, I learned never to assume anything. In the case of the wrong amputation, the chain of mistakes began with an orderly who had put the tag on the wrong leg, and nobody asked the patient which leg was to be amputated! If the nurse, the surgeon or the anesthesiologist had simply asked the patient, the mistake wouldn't have been made.

Looking back at Martha's case, I should have admitted her to the hospital. If her heart stopped, we could have performed CPR right there. Hindsight is always 20/20. We were all very fortunate that she had a quick-thinking husband.

Chapter 17
The Man from Shafter

IN THE SUMMER OF 1980, I was finally finished with all my training. I had arrived in the US in 1965, and fifteen years later I had passed all the examinations and was qualified to practice in every state in the US, as well as being board certified in ophthalmology.

I had thought about returning to Hong Kong to practice, but after a fact-finding visit, I learned that I would have to take their basic medical licensure. By then I was so tired of exams that I was in no mood to take another one, especially one that would only test my general medical knowledge instead of my specialty, ophthalmology.

In the end, I didn't sit for the Hong Kong medical licensure examination, deciding that my life was now in California and not Hong Kong. All my young life, I'd wanted to get away from Hong Kong for fear of the communists. It would make no sense for me to return, especially now that my parents had moved to the US, and I had no close relatives left there.

I hadn't really put too much thought into where I was going to practice because I was so busy during my training, but once I decided not to return to Hong Kong, I knew I would most likely stay in California.

Before Mary and I made the decision to stay in California, we did check out Hawaii just to convince ourselves that it was the right decision. I interviewed at the prestigious Straub Clinic in Honolulu and was discouraged to discover that the ophthalmologists there were working very hard and not getting paid as much as those in California, and that living expenses in Hawaii were higher. Another reason that dissuaded us was that many families chose to send their children to private schools, which would be a great expense for us, as by then we had three children. Even though I loved Hawaii, to work and live there with a young family would be another thing.

On my return to California, I took an offer in Bakersfield, a town about a two-hour drive from Fresno, and one that I knew very little about. In fact, I'd never been to Bakersfield except for the job interview.

Two months into my job, I realized that it was a mistake to have taken the position. My boss, Dr. Humphrey, was an eccentric man and a terrible surgeon, but he refused to accept his incompetence and continued to operate. Case after case, his patients' sight got worse after surgery. I decided that I couldn't be part of it and submitted my resignation.

My contract was for twelve months, so I had to finish the year. Since I had no training in setting up an office, I decided to spend my free time with the billing department and learn how to bill for my services and other aspects of running a private practice.

One Friday afternoon, a Chinese couple arrived at the clinic. The man had come in because the vision in his right eye had gone totally dark the day before. He was in his early or mid-fifties, slim, with hollow cheeks and jet-black hair combed backwards. He sounded educated when he spoke. His wife was perhaps a few years younger. They spoke Mandarin, which I also spoke.

An examination showed that he had an extensive retinal detachment in his right eye and needed surgery as soon as possible to prevent permanent loss of vision. He had severe myopia, which was a common cause of retinal detachment, because the eye was elongated and the retina and other tissues had been stretched thin.

I was very surprised when I learned that the couple lived in Shafter, a town about 20 miles northwest of Bakersfield, and owned a Chinese restaurant called the *Rice Bowl.*

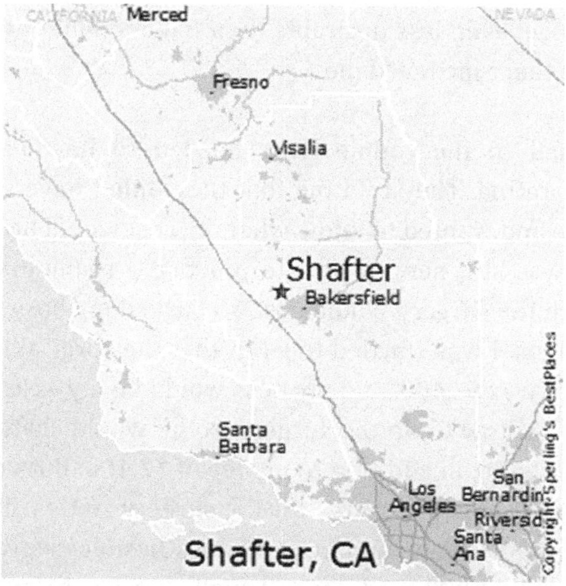

I wondered why these two seemingly educated people from Taiwan had settled in a town like Shafter. I'd heard a lot of jokes about the Bakersfield area on late-night shows, especially the Johnny Carson Show.

A week earlier, my friend Chuck and his family had driven down from Kingsburg to visit and show us his new van. The following morning, he found the entire van covered with brown oily droplets. It turned out that they were the precipitation from the oil refinery nearby in Oildale. I was told that poor quality oil like that from the Bakersfield area produced the droplets. I imagined these same oil droplets getting trapped in our lungs and causing severe health problems.

Since I'd moved to Bakersfield, I found my asthma had gotten worse, and I'd developed chronic bronchitis, which I ascribed to the pollution from the oil refinery as well as the spraying of all sorts of chemicals on the cotton and other crops.

Shafter was a farming community with a population of less than 15,000 in 1980. By any measure, it was not a very desirable place to live, even less desirable than Bakersfield. How the Lius ended up there intrigued me.

I explained to the couple what needed to be done for the detached retina. They told me that they didn't have any health insurance and wanted to know what the cost would be.

As I was still new to private practice, I really didn't know how much the surgery would cost, so I asked my boss to explain it to the Lius. I was startled to learn that the surgical fee for the procedure was $2,400, and my boss would be my assistant as he didn't know how to do the surgery, so he would charge 20% of $2,400, or $480, in addition to my fee of $2,400. But what really surprised me was the charge for the surgery suite, which would be over $6,000. We would need an anesthesiologist, who would cost around $1,000, and several nights at the hospital, which would be at least $1,000 a night. The total was $14,000 if everything went as planned.

I really felt bad for the couple. I apologized and said there was nothing I could do to reduce the cost because I was just an employee of the clinic.

Later in my own private practice, I would usually donate my services for those who didn't have any insurance, and tried to ask the anesthesiologist to reduce his or her fee. The hospital's fees were non-negotiable.

The surgery was a difficult one because Mr. Liu was really myopic and the sclera was extremely thin, which could lead to all sorts of complications. But it was successful and the retina was fully re-attached, and I discharged him in two days instead of the usual five days in order to save him some money.

The couple was grateful that in this remote part of America, they'd run into someone who spoke their language. Before leaving the hospital, they invited me to visit their restaurant.

Two months later, on a late Saturday afternoon, Mary and I and our three young children drove to Shafter. The Lius' restaurant was a small, old house that had been remodeled, with six tables. Mr. Liu was back working.

Mary and I checked out the menu and noted that each dish cost about $3 or $4. I thought about how many dishes this poor man had to cook to pay for his surgery. I felt bad.

Mr. Liu recommended stir-fry beef with asparagus, fried noodle, minced beef and egg white soup with cilantro, and fried chicken. The food was good.

When it was time to leave, I insisted on paying, but the Lius refused to take my money.

I wished we could've stayed longer because I was really curious about how they ended up in this area, but by then the kids were getting restless.

Before we left, I asked them if Mary and I could take them out to dinner on their day of rest, which was Tuesday.

Two weeks later, with a babysitter taking care of the children, we met up with Liu and his wife, Sally, at the Bamboo Garden in Bakersfield for dinner.

"How did you end up in Shafter?" I asked once we were settled at our table.

"We lived in LA for a couple of years and tried to make a living there," said Liu. "But there wasn't much we could do. We both majored in literature at university in Taiwan, so our credentials are useless in this country. We tried to open a restaurant, but with so many good chefs in the LA area, we simply couldn't compete," he lamented.

"How did you find out about Shafter?" I asked.

"I had a cousin who was working as an engineer in an oil refinery in Oildale, so we thought we would give this place a try," remarked Liu.

"How do you like it here?"

Sally answered. "Life is tough here because the people are mostly uneducated and few are wealthy," she commented. "As you know, most of them work in agriculture or oil. We feel very isolated because there are only three other Chinese families here.

"We'll never get rich, but we are making a living," she continued. "But I'm worried about our thirteen-year-old son Jason. He's learning bad habits from other kids. He talks back at us. When he was younger, we used to send him back to Taiwan in the summer to live with my parents, so he would at least get some Chinese culture—things such as respecting one's parents. But this year, he simply refused to go. We argued and we screamed, but in the end, there was nothing we could do to make him go to Taiwan," she sighed.

"It looked like you have a good business when we were there," I remarked.

Liu nodded his agreement. "The people in Shafter are generally nice. They're pleased that there's a Chinese restaurant in town, and they don't have to drive all the way to Bakersfield."

"Dr. Hung, you are so fortunate to be a doctor in America," said Sally. "Working in a Chinese restaurant is a hard way to make a living. When we were in university, we were so romantic and idealistic. We dreamed about living in Paris or Rome. We talked about walking along the Seine River in Paris or visiting the Trevi Fountain in Rome. Now, we are in the middle of nowhere, and it's so very hot in the summer," she lamented.

After the server came by to take our dinner order, I continued with my inquiries. "Why did you leave Taiwan?" I asked.

"You know, life is difficult in Taiwan," Sally replied. "Just as you worried about the communists taking over Hong Kong, we too worried about them invading Taiwan. We were worried about our son too because he would be drafted into the Taiwanese Army when he turned 18. So, when my brother became a US citizen, we applied for immigrant visas, and they were approved."

I nodded, understanding their desire to pursue a life in America, because it had been my dream too. "What do you do in your spare time?" I asked, changing the subject.

"What keeps us from going crazy are the books we brought along," Sally answered. "We both like literature and poetry. We both like to read as well as write Tang style poetry. It's amazing that the poems written almost a thousand years ago by poets like Li Bai, Du Fu or Wang Wei are still very relevant today."

"Dr. Hung, do you like Tang poetry?" asked Liu.

"I'm embarrassed to admit that my education was mostly a British one," I responded. "Yes, in Hong Kong I studied Chinese, but part of my life I spent in Malaysia and studied Malay and English. So my foundation of the Chinese language is really quite meager. But to answer your question, yes, I do, I know a few of the poems. But I don't know enough to compose anything similar."

The owner and chef of the Bamboo Garden was a fellow from Hong Kong. Mary and I had been to this restaurant on several occasions and I had gotten to know the forty-odd-year-old Ringo Tam. Usually when we went, we would tell Ringo just to cook a few dishes he thought we'd like. He had never disappointed us, and we especially liked the steamed fish.

On this occasion, Ringo came out of the kitchen to say hello to us. I introduced the Lius to Ringo and his wife, May, who was the cashier as well as a waitress.

The Tams were from Hong Kong and didn't speak Mandarin, and the Lius were from Taiwan, and they spoke no Cantonese, so it was difficult for them to communicate. I was very fortunate to have learnt both dialects when I was young.

During dinner, I again apologized to the Lius that I couldn't talk my boss into giving them a discount because I was just an employee, and explained that I would be leaving the area to set up my own practice in Fresno when my contract finished at the end of June.

As we were busy eating and talking, I noticed a couple enter the restaurant. The man had a blond, pompadour hairstyle, and the woman had a beehive hairstyle.

Ringo greeted them, "Good evening, Mr. and Mrs. Alan," and then passed by our table and commented that they were both country singers. I didn't recognize either of them.

"It seems these country western singers like Chinese food," I quipped.

"Yes, they do," Ringo remarked. "They're good people and are usually big tippers. They like our special deep fried whole chicken, as well as deep fried catfish fillets. For some reason, they also like our egg drop soup with tomato and tofu.

"I really like country music," Ringo continued. "In case you don't know, Buddy Alan is the son of Bonnie Campbell and Buck Owens, who was also a famous country singer. Buddy Alan's real name is Alan Edgar "Buddy" Owens. To make it more confusing, Bonnie Campbell (Buck Owens' former wife) later married another very famous country singer in the area."

It was interesting to learn about Bakersfield, and the many famous country western singers from the area.

"I do like country music, but my taste is quite restricted to just a few of the really old singers, such as Slim Whitman and

Hank Williams," I commented. "I don't appreciate Merle Haggard or the other Bakersfield area country singers' style. They're not smooth like Slim Whitman."

I'd learned that the Bakersfield sound was a sub-genre of country music developed in the mid to late 1950s in and around Bakersfield. It was the first style of country music significantly influenced by rock and roll, relying heavily on electric instrumentation.

"I also like country music," Ringo agreed. "The Nashville sound is thought of as a little bit more smooth, more polished, more refined, but I've learned to like the Bakersfield sound."

As Ringo and I talked about country music, the Lius were totally lost. They had no idea what we were talking about. Ringo headed back to the kitchen as more customers showed up.

We had a good dinner and a good visit. I told the Lius that we must meet again.

***

Even though my year at the Bakersfield eye clinic wasn't an ideal one, along the way I took care of interesting patients, met fascinating people and learned how to run a private practice. It was like an internship in the business part of a medical practice.

When my contract was up, we moved to Fresno at the end of June, 1981, where I opened my own private practice.

The year in Bakersfield was not lost. As I set up my practice, I appreciated how much I'd learned from the billing manager there, such as how much to charge for each procedure, something we never learned in medical school.

Life got busy and we never returned to the *Rice Bowl* or *Bamboo Garden*.

Now and then I would think of the Lius, wondering how they were doing in Shafter.

Chapter 18
Mrs. Zafrarini

I STILL FEEL BAD for what happened to Mrs. Zafrarini after all these years. It was a series of unfortunate circumstances that led to her unnecessary suffering.

In 1981, after all my years of training, I was excited to start my own practice in Fresno. In order to do surgeries at the hospital, a new doctor needed to apply for privileges. The new surgeon would be monitored by three staff members of the same specialty. Each time the new surgeon was to perform surgery, he or she had to call one of the monitors to be present so the surgery could be evaluated. One member of the staff would also go over every chart the new surgeon had written.

Being new in town, I was careful to obey all the rules and regulations; if anything, I was overly cautious.

Early on in my practice, money was scarce, so I tried to do things myself, like wiring the equipment in my new office. I even put in a sound system on my own.

To drum up referrals, I visited doctors in the area and gave lectures and workshops on Saturdays to optometrists in the San Joaquin Valley. I was pleased to see that almost all forty or so optometrists in the area showed up at every lecture and workshop. Before long, patients began calling for appointments.

One of the doctors I visited was Dr. Tong, who had trained at the Mayo clinic and whose father was Chinese and mother Jamaican. He took care of many diabetic patients. Soon, he was referring all his patients with eye problems to me.

One patient Dr. Tong referred to me was Mrs. Zafrarini. She was a beautiful woman, about seventy years old, with porcelain skin and light brown hair always perfectly coiffured. Her son was Dr. Tong's CPA and financial adviser. She was unhappy with the ophthalmologist she was seeing, and so she ended up in my office.

Mrs. Zafrarini had been diagnosed with diabetes in her twenties and since then had been giving herself daily injections of insulin. As I took her history, she revealed that she'd had laser treatment in her left eye by a doctor who had a bad reputation for doing procedures he wasn't trained in, and after the treatment her vision got a lot worse. She was never told why.

As I examined her, I saw evidence of the poorly done laser treatment, but what devastated me was the macula (central vision), which had been destroyed by a laser burn. Treating the macula by mistake was one of the potential complications of laser treatment, as trying to view the inside of the eye took experience. Sometimes the surgeon "got lost" or disoriented with the landmarks inside the eye, not realizing that the macula was being treated. I was certain that's what happened to Mrs. Zafrarini.

There was some bleeding in her right (untreated) eye, and I told her that at some point the right eye would need laser treatment as well.

"Dr. Hung, what happened to my left eye?" she asked. "Why did my vision get so much worse after the laser treatment?"

Not ready to tell her the bad news, I told her that scarring had caused the loss of vision. In a way it was true, because it was the scarring caused by the laser burn that had destroyed the macula, and hence caused the loss of her central vision.

After Mrs. Zafrafini left, I called Dr. Tong and explained the unfortunate situation to him. He was literally speechless. In fact,

I had to ask him if he was still on the phone because of the long silence.

Dr. Tong felt devastated because it was he who'd referred Mrs. Zafrarini to this other doctor, and not only was Mrs. Zafrarini his patient, but her son was also his very good friend.

It turned out that this foreign-trained doctor had tried to take the Ophthalmology Board Exam five times, and he failed each time. The training he had in his home country didn't include laser treatment.

To make things worse, Mrs. Zafrarini's son's office was next to Dr. Tong's, and so was this doctor's office.

I asked Dr. Tong if he thought I should tell Mrs. Zafrarini the truth. He replied that since it was he who'd referred her, he would talk to her son and see if he wanted to take any action against the other doctor.

It was now October in 1981. My practice was growing, and I was also traveling to Madera, a town twenty miles north of Fresno, for half a day each week to see patients with retinal problems. In addition, I was also traveling to Merced, a town 50 miles north of Fresno, for another half day every week for consultations.

It was stressful being a new surgeon in town, as there were so many things to tend to.

In early November, I saw Mrs. Zafrarini again. The situation with her left eye wasn't brought up—it seemed that Dr. Tong hadn't discussed the issue with her son.

Now, her right eye showed areas of new vessels growing and needing laser treatment. If left untreated, these new vessels would bleed or become fibrous tissue and pull on the retina, causing the retina to detach—a condition called traction retinal detachment.

Usually, the treatment—called PRP (Pan Retinal Photocoagulation)—wasn't difficult, and I'd done hundreds of them during my residency and fellowship. However, being new in town and considering Mrs. Zafrarini's very delicate situation, I decided to refer her to my mentor at UCSF where I'd done my retinal surgery fellowship. Professor Maxwell was a big name in the retina circle. He had pioneered and developed many surgical procedures, and had written several books on retinal surgery.

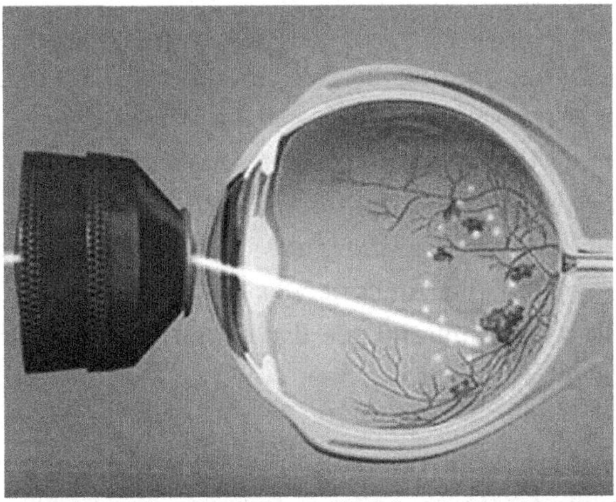

Laser Photocoagulation of Diabetic Retinopathy

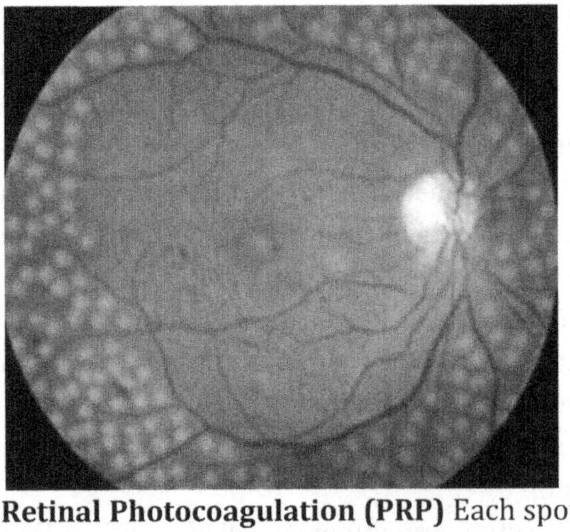

After Pan Retinal Photocoagulation (PRP) Each spot is a laser treatment spot. The macula (central vision) is in the center. The optic nerve is on the right, where the blood vessels originate.

A few days before Thanksgiving, I began to feel like my balance was off. In the office, I had to put my hands on the wall to walk so I wouldn't fall down. Something was obviously wrong, but I chose to ignore it.

When I tried to start my car and had to use both hands on the ignition because they were so weak, I knew something was really wrong.

The day before Thanksgiving, I found myself gasping for air. Mary drove me to the hospital and I was promptly admitted. Initially the neurologist didn't know what was causing my issues, so they ran tests to rule out a brain tumor.

When the imaging studies showed no tumor, they did a spinal tap and made the diagnosis of Guillain-Barre Syndrome, an autoimmune condition most likely related to stress.

I was admitted to the ICU and put on a ventilator. In spite of being totally paralyzed, I had horrible pain all over my body and was given a morphine drip to alleviate the pain.

While I was in the ICU, Mrs. Zafrarini had gone up to see Dr. Maxwell and he did laser treatment in her right eye.

On her return to Fresno, she told her son that the vision in her right eye was really bad and she could no longer read. Her son called my office.

By now, my illness was the talk of the medical community, how this young doctor, just finished all his training and barely four months into his practice, was barely clinging on to life. I had developed severe pneumonia in both lungs, and the prognosis for my survival was 50/50.

All the ophthalmologists in Fresno got together to help cover my patients—not that I had very many at that point. Mrs. Zafrarini was referred to another retinal specialist who belonged to one of the two large specialist groups in the area.

From my past experience with Dr. Finley, I'd found him to be a passive aggressive sort of man. He was in his mid-forties and was always complaining about other doctors.

After he'd examined Mrs. Zafrarini, he began ranting that the doctor in San Francisco had done too much laser, and now the vision was affected because there was a great deal of edema in the retina.

"Why did Dr. Hung send you up to San Francisco?" he asked Mrs. Zarfarini and her son. "I could have done a much better job here. The doctor in San Francisco did too much laser at one time, and it caused a lot of swelling in your retina, which is why your vision is so blurry."

Mrs. Zafrarini and her son were understandably upset and confused. They knew that I had nothing to gain by sending her to the top retina doctor in the country. The son called my office and asked what they should do.

As I lay motionless in the ICU with a tube in my trachea connected to a ventilator, in constant pain, I was in no shape to make any decisions. Mary told Mrs. Zafrarini's son to call Dr. Maxwell and let him know what was happening.

It was a long drive to San Francisco, and Mrs. Zafrarini wondered if there was another retina specialist in town. Dr. Maxwell suggested the other retina doctor from the second large group of local specialists.

Dr. Don was a retired Navy Admiral and was well respected in town. He was kind and took time to examine Mrs. Zafrarini, telling her that swelling of the retina was one of the side effects of laser treatment, and that in most cases it would get better with time.

Over the following months, her vision did improve, but never returned to the level it was before the treatment. However, the laser treatment had stopped the proliferation of new blood vessels, preventing the eye from bleeding or having a detached retina.

After almost a month in the ICU, and another month in the hospital, I gradually improved. With physical therapy, I learned to walk again. I had to relearn to talk and how to do basic things like doing up a button.

In April of the following year, I was well enough to return to work. Mrs. Zafrarini was one of the first patients I saw when I got back into the office. She was as graceful as ever.

When she saw me, she gave me a big hug and had tears in her eyes, saying how happy she was to see me back at work.

I never found out if Dr. Tong told Mrs. Zafrarini or her son about the accidental treatment of the left macula by the foreign-trained doctor. If they'd decided to sue that doctor, they could have a case, but Mrs. Zafrarini didn't seem like someone who would sue.

Over the years, Mrs. Zafrarini needed additional laser treatments, which I was able to do in my office.

As she got older, her long history of diabetes began to exact more of a toll on her aging body, and eventually her kidneys began to fail. I visited her at the hospital when she was being evaluated for hemodialysis. In spite of her poor vision, she still managed to put on her makeup, and she still looked elegant.

A few years later, Mrs. Zafrarini passed away at age 80.

Because of the lessons I learned from her, I always made sure that I didn't over-treat a patient's eye. Just like taking medicine, if you take too much, you can't undo what you've already consumed. If you don't take enough, you can always add more later. I kept that in mind with every treatment I did.

My policy for laser treatment was to do it in three sessions, about two weeks apart, so there wouldn't be too much swelling or any damage from the heat of the laser.

I will always have very fond memories of Mrs. Zafrarini, but at the same time I feel bad that she had to suffer the unnecessary loss of vision in her left eye through the incompetence of one doctor. I've debated with myself many times whether I should have told her the truth about her left eye. In the end, I felt that I did the right thing to refer her to my mentor, thinking that his authority made him the best person to explain what had happened. But unfortunately, instead of helping Mrs. Zafrarini, another complication arose. Medicine can be unpredictable, and sometimes things just happen.

I remind myself that we should learn from our mistakes or experiences and move on. It doesn't help to continue to beat ourselves up. We're only human.

Chapter 19

Julia Norberg

JULIA NORBERG WAS NINETEEN YEARS OLD when I first met her. She had a soft face with a perfect nose and a shy smile. She reminded me of Ingrid Bergman, one of my favorite actresses, whom I'd discovered in the movie *Casablanca*. Like Ingrid Bergman, Julia wore little or no makeup. She had natural beauty. Her hair was light brown like Ingrid Bergman's, but her large eyes were hazel instead of Ingrid's blue. She also had a build similar to the actress's, with broad shoulders and a boyish torso.

She was referred to me by her endocrinologist, Dr. Warren Mason, the only fellowship-trained endocrinologist in the San Joaquin Valley at the time. Julia had Type I diabetes, which was diagnosed when she was eight years old.

Her family was originally from St. Paul, Minnesota and both parents were of Swedish descent. Her father was an engineer who was transferred to Tennessee, where Julia was born and grew up.

She spoke with a slight southern accent, which seemed a little incongruous with her northern European look. After high school, she moved to be near her brother, who was two years older than her and was stationed at the Lemoore Naval Air Station, not far from Fresno.

Julia attended the California State University Fresno—just Fresno State to most people—majoring in Business Administration. She also worked part time as a receptionist at the Holiday Inn by the airport.

Dr. Mason referred most of his diabetic patients to me, because after years with the disease, many of them would develop retinopathy. If detected early, the treatment was easy and safe and the laser treatment was easily done in the office. However, if detected late, after damage had been done, the loss of vision usually couldn't be reversed.

After examining Julia's eyes, I noted that, indeed, she had the beginning of diabetic retinopathy; but it wasn't yet serious enough to require treatment.

As with all my young female patients who had diabetes, I warned her about the risks of getting pregnant, because during pregnancy a diabetic woman's hormones increase tremendously.

Estrogen and progesterone are the chief pregnancy hormones. A woman will produce more estrogen during one pregnancy than throughout her entire life when not pregnant. The increase in estrogen during pregnancy enables the uterus and placenta to improve vascularization, i.e. the formation of blood vessels. The formation of new blood vessels in the eye can cause bleeding, or when these vessels mature and form scars, they can pull the retina off.

Pregnancy can worsen certain long-term diabetes problems, such as eye problems and kidney disease, especially if one's blood glucose levels are too high.

There is also a greater chance of developing preeclampsia, sometimes called toxemia, which is when one develops high blood pressure and too much protein in the urine during the second half of pregnancy. Preeclampsia can cause serious or life-threatening problems for the mother and the baby.

Julia listened to my explanation and advice carefully and asked some pertinent questions. She seemed like a responsible young woman who had a great future ahead of her in spite of her diabetes.

Because of her retinopathy, I asked her to return in three months for a reevaluation.

After she left, I recalled my own college days, and how at nineteen I was confused and often lost, not knowing which direction my life should go. In contrast, Julia had a plan and her future seemed bright.

When she returned three months later, Julia brought her brother Paul with her. He was in his navy uniform, and was a very handsome young man with a strong resemblance to his sister. They seemed very close.

During the examination, I noted that Julia's retinopathy had progressed and I suggested doing a fluorescein angiogram. Fluorescein Angiography (FA) is a diagnostic procedure that uses a special camera to record the blood flow in the retina, and to get a better look at the blood vessels and other structures in the back of the eye.

I was concerned, because in just three months there had been noticeable changes in her retina.

"How is your blood sugar and blood pressure?" I asked.

"Dr. Hung, it's not easy going to school and working at the same time," Julia replied, "let alone trying to check my blood sugar several times a day. Dr. Mason thinks I'm not doing a good job with checking my blood sugar. I think he's a little upset with me," she admitted.

"Julia, you're a young woman with many decades ahead of you. You must make it your priority to take care of your health and prevent the complications that can come with diabetes, especially since you've had it since you were eight," I remarked.

"Yes, I know. I'll try," she responded.

"Let me show you what I found in your eyes," I said, and then showed her the fluorescein angiogram as well as the color pictures of her eyes.

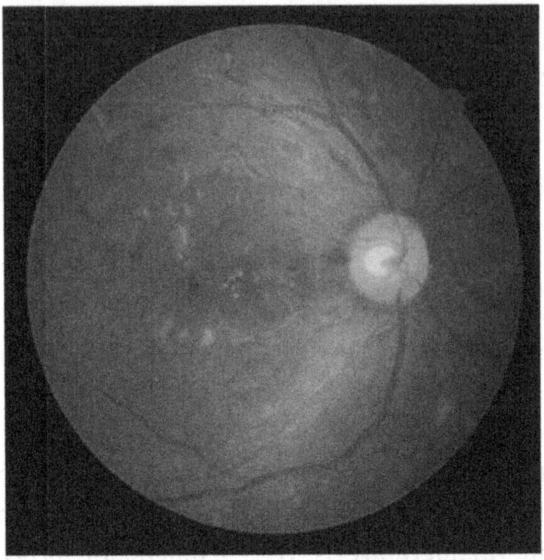

Diabetic retinopathy with bleeding in multiple areas.

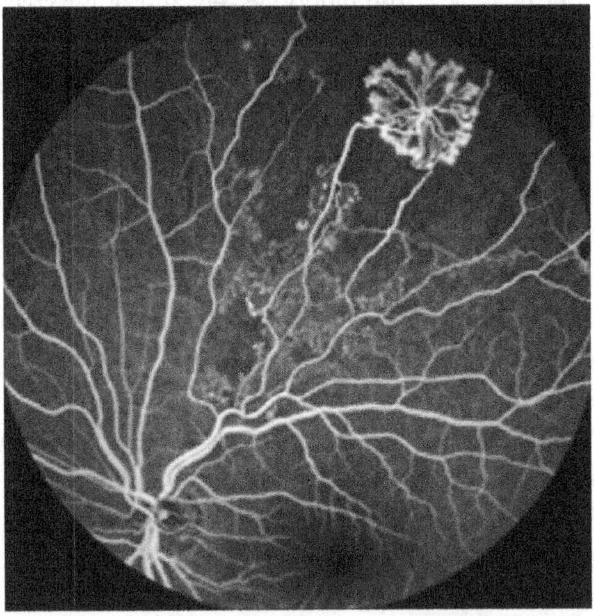

New vessels are growing in the upper right-hand corner in this fluorescein angiogram.

I pointed out the differences between the initial color pictures and the ones from that day's visit as well as the fluorescein angiogram, which showed an area of new vessels—called a neovascular frond in proliferative diabetic retinopathy.

"These new vessels are unlike normal blood vessels," I explained. "They're more prone to leak or rupture, and when that happens it can fill the eye with blood. If there's blood in the eye, you can't see. If these new vessels aren't treated, and even if they don't bleed, eventually they can cause scar formation and pull on the retina, which can cause a condition called traction retinal detachment. If that happens, it can make your eye go blind."

I pointed to an area on the angiogram. "Today, I suggest that we treat this nest of new vessels. It will take about 15 minutes. It's not a big area, and most likely won't be painful," I added.

Her brother Paul had been listening, and nodded. Julia agreed.

My assistant put a few anesthetic drops in Julia's left eye, and seated her in front of the laser machine.

I placed a special large contact lens on her eye, and focused the laser beam to the area of new vessels. After applying about 200 spots placed on and surrounding the new vessels, I stopped.

"That should do it," I said.

"Thank you. That wasn't bad," Julia exclaimed.

Paul put his right arm around his sister's shoulders as they entered the waiting room to make another appointment to return in a month. I wanted to see her sooner than usual because I was surprised how much the retinopathy had progressed in the previous three months.

When she returned the next month, I was relieved to find no noticeable change.

After that, I would see Julia every three months or so. I always enjoyed her visits, as she reminded me of my own youth, and I truly liked her. I felt that she also liked me as her doctor—she always seemed happy to see me and greeted me with a warm smile.

She wasn't a loquacious person and was often a little shy, only speaking when I asked her questions.

"How's school?" I asked on one visit.

"I'm taking some time off because I was stressed out with both the work and the school," she replied.

"How's your blood sugar?" I asked.

"It's still not ideal," she admitted. "Dr. Mason seems to be having a tough time getting it under control. In fact, he says he's going to put an insulin pump on me," she added.

"Good," I said with a nod of approval. "I hope that makes it easier for you."

We continued on with our regular check-ups and visits for a year and a half. During that time, I had to do more laser treatments in both of her eyes. Her vision remained 20/20, and she wasn't having any problems with night-time driving like some other patients who'd had extensive laser treatments.

She often wrote notes to me, thanking me for taking good care of her, saying that she appreciated my patience listening to her concerns and that she knew I truly cared for her wellbeing.

When she didn't show up for one of her appointments, I was worried. There was no news from her. My assistant tried to contact her, but she didn't answer. I called Dr. Mason to ask if he'd seen Julia and he replied that he hadn't seen her in over six months.

With her labile blood sugar and blood pressure, in addition to her retinopathy, I was worried. I thought about calling her brother, but I hesitated because during that time there was a lot of talk in the media about patient privacy rights.

I'd also learned a hard lesson about it two years earlier. One of the deans at Fresno State University had been referred to me for bleeding in the eye. It turned out to be a vein occlusion. I followed him closely. He always came alone, and was always quiet, rarely acknowledging if he understood the seriousness of his condition.

As a concerned doctor, I thought his family should know. I called his home, and when his wife answered, I told her about the dean's situation. She said she would talk to him about seeing his internist to evaluate if his blood was normal.

The following day, this dean called me on the phone, saying that I had violated his privacy by telling his wife about his condition without his permission. He was really upset.

I was dumbfounded. I thought I was being a good doctor with good communication. I truly had no idea why he was so angry. I later I learned that I had indeed violated his right to privacy.

Two days later, the optometrist who had referred him to me called and said that the dean had chastised him also, and that he and his family would no longer go to him because he'd referred him to a doctor who didn't respect his privacy.

To this day, I've never understood why he was so angry with me. I knew that there must be a hidden agenda or some reasonable explanation, but I had no idea what.

A month later, I read in the local paper that the dean has died of a stroke while on a cruise to Mexico. It turned out that he had some sort of leukemia and his blood was thick, which was why he had the vein occlusion.

Because of that experience, I decided not to call Julia's brother.

A few days before Christmas Julia showed up in my office. She had called earlier in the day and told my receptionist that she needed to see me as soon as possible.

When I walked into the examination room, I hardly recognized her. Her face was all puffy, and I could tell she'd been crying. She looked very sad and seemed distraught.

As soon as she saw me, she got up, flung her arms around me and started crying. I was startled.

"What's the matter?" I asked in a concerned voice.

"Dr. Hung, I've been so stupid," she sniffled. "I've made a mess of my life. I don't know what to do. Maybe you can give me some advice, because Dr. Mason is really mad at me."

"Please sit down," I said kindly, guiding her to a chair. I pulled a stool up and sat next to her, gently patting her right knee. "Tell me what happened."

"I was such a fool," she said tearfully. "I fell in love with one of the assistant managers at the Holiday Inn. We talked about marriage. We talked about moving to Portland where he was from. Then I got pregnant. We went to Portland, but neither of us had a job. One day, he just disappeared. I didn't know what to do. I was too ashamed to tell my parents. My brother Paul came to Portland to help me. In the meantime, I neglected my insulin. One day, I got up and my face was all puffy and my left eye was completely dark.

"Finally, I called my parents," she continued. "They came out to Portland to help me move back to Fresno so you and Dr. Mason could continue to take care of me. But Dr. Mason is really mad at me because he said I didn't take his advice and it would be very difficult for him to take care of me. My parents pleaded with him, and he finally agreed to continue helping manage my disease.

"I'm really worried about my eyes," she cried. "All those complications you told me about on the first visit seem to have come true. It's entirely my own fault. I was so stupid," she finished with a sob.

"Julia, when we're young, we make mistakes. I made my fair share of them when I was your age," I said, trying to console her.

I sat with her until she regained her composure, and then said, "Now, let's see what's going on with your eyes."

After dilating Julia's pupils, I examined her carefully. The left eye was filled with blood. I did an ultrasound scan on her and fortunately found no detached retina. Her right eye had 20/40 vision, but had multiple areas of new vessels.

"The vision in your right eye is still good," I explained. "But it needs more laser right away. You left eye is filled with blood, which may go away on its own. If it doesn't, we can do a surgery called vitrectomy to remove it."

Once I was caught up with my regular patients, I did an extensive laser treatment on her right eye. "I'm quite sure we'll be able to maintain the vision in the right eye," I reassured Julia and her parents.

Julia's parents were in their early fifties, and seemed like genuinely kind people. Aside, her mother said to me, "Dr. Hung, Julia has talked about you so much. She thinks you are the most wonderful doctor in the world."

I smiled and replied, "Julia is a good girl. I really like her. She's young, and I told her that we all make mistakes sometimes."

After the Norbergs left, I called Dr. Mason to tell him the condition of Julia's eyes. By then, Dr. Mason had calmed down and said that he was sorry he'd lost patience with Julia. He'd been frustrated because by disappearing for six months, her body went to hell. All the dreaded complications occurred. Her kidney function was now only 20%, which explained why her face was so puffed up. It might not be long before she needed renal dialysis.

With her parents' help, Julia returned to Fresno State and found a studio apartment one block from the university.

Six months later, the blood in Julia's left eye remained dense. I suggested that a vitrectomy be performed to remove the blood and recommended more laser treatment if necessary to prevent further bleeding. Her mother again flew from Tennessee to help take care of her following the surgery.

Everything went well. While inside the eye, I removed some scar tissue caused by maturation of the new vessels, and I did more laser treatment.

Julia was now seeing a nephrologist and he told her that she would soon need dialysis. A month later, she came by the office to say goodbye.

"My mother decided that she would donate one of her kidneys to me," she said. "The surgery will be done at Vanderbilt University Medical Center. Can you give the name of a retina specialist in Tennessee?"

"Dr. Steve Charles is in fact the world's most famous retina specialist, and he happens to be in Memphis," I replied. "I'll have my assistant get his address and phone number for you. She'll also prepare your records for you to take to him."

I was sad to see Julia go, but she promised to keep in touch, and she made good on that promise. She had a successful kidney transplant, and Dr. Charles' associates did more laser treatment in both of her eyes.

Her parents bought her a small house in Johnson City, Tennessee, where East Tennessee State University was situated.

Julia wrote to me regularly. She graduated from Tennessee State University in library science instead of business administration and was working as a librarian at the university. She wrote that her brother became a pilot and that she was very proud of him.

I always looked forward to getting her letters, written in her beautiful penmanship.

She said that life was satisfactory and she had a nice circle of friends. It was good to be near her parents and some cousins.

Even though I'm a retina surgeon, I learned early on that the specialist shouldn't only treat the part of the body in which he or she specializes. We must treat the patient as a whole human being. I think Julia liked me because she could feel that I was concerned not only about her eyes, but about her as a person.

One of the greatest satisfactions in being a physician is to know your patients understand that you care about them and try to do your best for them.

Julia was very fortunate to have such a loving family who came to her rescue when she made a mistake. We are all human, and we all make mistakes.

Chapter 20
The Nurse's Son

IT WAS LATE ON A FRIDAY AFTERNOON. We were almost finished seeing patients when Debbie Hudson, the head nurse in the surgery department of the nearby hospital, showed up with a young man.

Her 24-year-old son Jon had been working on the construction of a large home in a gated community with its own artificial lake in north Fresno. He was struck in the eye by a staple from a staple gun. Staple guns use a system of compressed air, which can rapidly and powerfully shoot staples into wood.

Jon was immediately seen by Dr. Shuman, head of the Occupational Medicine Clinic that took care of most of the workman's comp cases in the San Joaquin Valley. He noted the injury and put an eye shield over it to protect the eye, and then referred Jon to my office. Dr. Shuman regularly referred his patients with eye injuries to me.

Jon was quiet and seemed dazed. He was a tall, handsome, muscular young man with shoulder-length dark blond hair and dark blue eyes. He told me that he was trying to hurry at the end of his shift, as he was planning to go out with some friends after work. He was loading a cartridge of staples when it accidently discharged. One staple hit him in the left eye. He felt a sharp pain and his vision became blurry.

His mother, who was at home at the time, immediately drove to Dr. Shuman's office, picked Jon up and brought him to my office.

I gently removed the blue plastic eye shield and examined Jon's left eye. It was slightly red, and there was a little blood inside the eye in front of the pupil.

Covering his right eye, I asked him if he could see my fingers. The vision in his left eye was so blurry that he could only see my fingers at four feet.

I gently touched his eye with a sterile cotton tip applicator and noted that the eye was a little soft. I decided to do a Seidel test, which assesses if there's any leakage from the eyeball. A positive test would indicate leakage of aqueous humor from the anterior chamber, which would require immediate action.

I opened a sterile fluorescein strip and applied it to the areas of suspected leakage, then examined it with a cobalt blue filter. I noted green fluid slowly spreading from about the 3 o'clock position, just as I had suspected. The test was positive and confirmed a small leak in Jon's eye. This was an ocular emergency.

First, we needed to make sure that the injured eye didn't get infected. I told Debbie that her son needed to be admitted to the hospital for IV antibiotics.

Before sending Jon to the hospital, thankfully only half a block away, I told Debbie that the leak had to be sealed, and we could do it with Super Glue.

During my fellowship at UCSF, one of my research projects involved the use of Super Glue in retinal surgery, and I'd subsequently published a seminal paper in the *Ophthalmology Journal* about my findings.

Super Glue's scientific name is Cyanoacrylate, which is a family of strong, fast-acting adhesives. They're used in industrial, medical and household applications, and are sometimes known generically as instant glues, power glues, crazy glue or superglues.

I told Debbie that I was familiar with the use of Super Glue in eye injuries and surgeries, and reassured her that the glue was only temporary. I explained that Jon had developed a cataract caused by the staple, and it would need to be removed after we were certain the eye wasn't infected.

I got a small tube of the sterile glue from our fridge. After drying the area with a sterile cotton tip applicator, I applied it to the wound, noting that it adhered to the surface of the cornea where the leak was. After a few minutes, I again gently touched Jon's eye with a sterile cotton tip applicator, and noted that it was no longer soft, meaning that it was no longer leaking fluid.

The most important thing at that point was to make sure the eye didn't get infected. Unlike other organs, an infected eye was difficult to treat and could even result in loss of the eye.

I placed the shield back up to cover Jon's eye, wrote orders on the hospital admission form and ordered the IV antibiotics.

Debbie then drove Jon to the nearby St. Agnes Hospital where she worked. As they left, I told them I would join them shortly and go over treatment plans with them.

When I finished with my last patient for the day, I made the very short drive to St. Agnes and found Debbie and Jon anxiously waiting for me in the hospital room.

Looking at Jon, I said, "I know you're quite sure the staple didn't enter your eye, but I still have to make sure that a part of it didn't break off. If there's a piece of metal in your eye, the treatment would be very different. We would have to get it out. If there's no metal in your eye, then we can wait and make sure there's no infection, and then remove the cataract. So, the next step is to have an X-ray of the orbit," I explained.

Once the X-ray was done, I could see there was no sign of any metal inside Jon's eye. I examined Jon's eye again and was satisfied that the glue was doing its job sealing the wound, as when I again touched the eyeball with the sterile cotton tip applicator, it was definitely not soft like it was when I first saw him.

I delivered the good news and went over the treatment plan with Jon and Debbie. If there was no sign of infection by Monday, we would plan to remove the cataract on Tuesday. I also needed to know the status of the retina in Jon's left eye and would need to do an ultrasound to make sure there was no detached retina.

"Do you wear glasses?" I asked Jon.

"I have a pair of glasses, but I usually wear contact lens," he replied.

"Do both eyes have the same prescription?" I asked.

"I'm not sure. I think so," he answered.

I asked him that question because if we could take out his cataract the following week, we should consider placing an intraocular lens. In order to know what sort of power of IOL to put in, we had to do measurements. But with the injured eye, it might not be safe to put a solid probe directly on his cornea. If both eyes were the same, then we could measure the right eye and be quite sure that the left eye would need the same power of correction.

"I'll call his optometrist's office on Monday, and will let you know," Debbie offered.

The following day, I visited Jon at the hospital. There was no sign of any infection. The cataract, however, had gotten worse, and was now totally white and opaque.

"So far, so good," I reported. "There's no sign of infection. The cataract has gotten worse, but that doesn't change our plan."

I visited Jon again on Sunday morning. His mother was there.

"There's still no sign of infection," I observed. "If the eye was going to get infected, it would have done so by now. As long as nothing changes by tomorrow, we can go ahead and remove the cataract on Tuesday. Some surgeons would suggest just removing the cataract, and when it's healed an IOL could be put in, or you could continue wearing your contact lenses.

"My recommendation is to put the IOL in when we do the cataract surgery. That would save you from another surgery, and it's also the safest and easiest time to put the IOL in," I explained further. I told them to think about the options and let me know what they wanted to do.

I stopped in at the hospital early Monday morning to see Jon and said that I'd like to see him in my office, because the hospital didn't have an ophthalmic ultrasound machine to check on his retina, and they also didn't have the equipment to measure his eye for the power of the IOL.

At noon, Debbie drove Jon over to my office.

I set Jon up at the ultrasound machine and gently placed the probe over his left eyelids. He seemed more relaxed today. The ultrasound showed no sign of any detached retina or blood inside the eye.

"Oh, Dr. Hung, I called Jon's optometrist earlier and he gave me Jon's prescription for his glasses," Debbie announced, handing me a piece of paper showing that Jon's prescription was minus 2 myopic and both eyes were the same.

"Good," I responded with a nod. "We can measure his good eye and use that to calculate the power of the IOL for the left eye.

"Things are falling into place," I said. "We can do the surgery tomorrow, and put in the IOL if you want me to. This is my recommendation. It's what I would do in your situation. But I know people have different opinions and other considerations. If you don't want the IOL tomorrow, I understand. If you wish to have a second opinion, it would be perfectly fine with me. There's definitely time for a second opinion. Debbie, since you're the head nurse in surgery and know all the ophthalmologists in town, I'm sure you could get Jon into an office this afternoon," I added.

"Dr. Hung, I like your idea of an IOL," Jon said.

Debbie nodded in agreement. "Dr. Hung, I've worked with you for over ten years. You have a good reputation as an excellent, conscientious and careful surgeon. There's no need for a second opinion. I like your recommendation too."

As Tuesday was a regular surgery day, I already had several cases scheduled. Jon's surgery was to follow the last case, which would be about 3 pm.

"That would work for me," I remarked. "I'll re-schedule my afternoon patients."

Debbie then took Jon back to the hospital to continue his IV antibiotics.

That evening, as with all my surgical cases, I reviewed the steps and had in my mind exactly what I was going to do. Then I made drawings and notes detailing the steps of Jon's surgery.

The following day, the surgery began promptly at 3 pm.

I first removed the small piece of glue. Then, with a diamond blade, I entered the anterior chamber and enlarged the wound with a pair of micro-scissors. The cataract was now fluffy and soft. The anterior capsule of Jon's natural lens had been punctured—most likely by the staple. The now swollen lens had enlarged the tear in the anterior capsule.

With a low rate·of suction, I gently aspirated out the now very soft cataract. I didn't even have to use the ultrasound (phaco-emulsification) machine, which we usually did for more mature cataracts.

The entire cataract was removed in less than ten minutes. I then gingerly placed the IOL within the capsular bag of the remaining natural lens. It looked secure. The wound was then closed with several 10-O gauge black nylon sutures. And the surgery was finished.

I visited Jon early the next morning and removed his eye shield. The cornea of the left eye looked clear, and there was a red reflex, indicating that the vitreous was clear and the retina was attached. Jon was comfortable and relaxed.

I covered this right eye and asked, "What can you see?"

Jon was beaming. "Wow, this is really clear!" he exclaimed. "I can see the hands of the clock on the wall."

Shortly after, he was discharged from the hospital and Debbie took him home.

The next day, I examined him again in the office. His vision was 20/30. There was still a trace of edema in his cornea.

When he returned with his mother the following Monday, the vision in his left eye without any correction (glasses or contact lens) was 20/20.

"This is the best I've ever seen in my life," Jon said. "This means I don't have to wear my contact lenses anymore. This is amazing. I thought I was going to lose my eye, and now, this eye sees better than the other," he exclaimed.

Debbie was relieved. "Thank you so much, Dr. Hung," she said. "We truly appreciate your care and letting us know what you were thinking along the way. This has turned out so much better than I expected."

As Debbie and Jon were leaving the room, Debbie turned around and, with tears in her eyes, gave me a hug. "Thank you so much Dr. Hung," she repeated.

I've always believed that being a doctor is about solving your patient's problem(s). Sometimes there's more than one way to solve the problem and we must include our patients in the decision-making process.

One of the greatest joys of being a doctor is, of course, that your patient has turned out well and that you've made a difference in his or her life. But it's also important that they know you truly care about them.

Chapter 21

Elena Caballero

I MET ELENA CABALLERO more than 30 years ago, and since that time, we've never forgotten each other.

She was referred to me at my Fresno practice in 1988. She came from the nearby farming town of Sanger and worked as a farm worker in the San Joaquin Valley. She picked oranges during the winter, and peaches, apricots, plums and tomatoes during the summer.

She was 26 when I met her, a warm, compact woman just over five feet tall, with thick, jet-black hair down to her shoulders. She wore a pair of dark sunglasses and was in obvious discomfort, complaining that the light really bothered her, and both her head and eyes were hurting.

She had a two-week history of pain, redness, photophobia and blurring of vision in both eyes. There was associated history of tinnitus and vertigo. She had malaise, fever, headache, nausea and abdominal pain, but no stiffness of the neck or back. There were a few areas of loss of pigment on and around her eyelids but her eyelashes were normal. Examination of her hair revealed a few patches of gray.

There was no history of joint pain, and no history of oral ulceration. There was no backache and no history of cough, night sweats or chest pain. She had no prior history of ocular injury and no previous eye surgery. She was neither diabetic nor hypertensive. There was no family history of any eye disease except that her grandfather had cataract surgery at seventy.

Her vision was so bad that she could only see my fingers at a distance of four feet. Examination of her eyes showed severe bilateral inflammation inside her eyes (uveitis). Examination of her retinas showed diffused edema.

As I'd treated this sort of disease during my residency and fellowship, I easily made the diagnosis of Vogt-Koyanagi-Harada (VKH) disease.

VKH disease is a rare autoimmune inflammatory disorder of unknown origin that affects many body systems, including the eyes, ears, skin and meninges (the covering of the brain and spinal cord). The most noticeable symptom is a rapid loss of vision.

It was first described independently by three different doctors: Drs. Vogt, Koyanagi and Harada, as bilateral uveitis, exudative retinal detachments, integumentary disorders and neurologic abnormalities. It has an immune-genetic predisposition that's common in certain ethnic groups, appearing more often in Asian, Middle Eastern, Hispanic and Native American populations. Gender also plays a role—women are twice as likely as men to be affected by VKH.

I immediately put Elena on large doses of oral prednisone as well as intensive topical steroidal and dilating drops to keep her pupils open and prevent the irises from forming adhesions to the lens, which could result from the severe inflammation caused by the disease. If not treated soon enough, these adhesions could be permanent and cause the pupil to be misshaped.

Even with the large doses of oral prednisone, it was difficult to control her disease.

Steroid drugs, such as prednisone, work by lowering the activity of the immune system. Prednisone is used to treat many conditions, including hormonal disorders, skin diseases, arthritis, lupus, psoriasis, allergic conditions, ulcerative colitis,

Crohn's disease, eye diseases, lung diseases, asthma, tuberculosis, blood cell disorders, kidney disorders, leukemia, lymphoma, multiple sclerosis, and in organ transplant to prevent rejection. It's a powerful drug, but one that comes with many side effects.

In spite of being on large doses of prednisone, Elena's condition only improved slightly after the first week. I was worried about keeping her on the steroid long term, because one of the dreaded complications was avascular necrosis of the hip, which could debilitate the patient. The reason is unknown, but one hypothesis is that corticosteroids can increase lipid levels in our blood, reducing blood flow.

So, I decided to add another drug: cyclosporine. I had to work with her internist to start her on this drug, as it's another very powerful drug, commonly used in organ transplants to prevent rejection. It belongs to a group of medicines known as immunosuppressive agents. It can cause serious side effects, such as kidney problems, and it may also decrease the body's ability to fight infection. Elena's internist would do weekly blood tests and examine her for any such side effects.

I understood that both drugs were powerful and had many side effects, but Elena's disease was wreaking havoc in her body, and I simply had to stop her body from attacking itself, including destroying her eyes.

Fortunately, after six months of close follow-up, seeing her sometimes twice a week, and slowly reducing the dosage of her medications, her disease quieted down and she didn't suffer any serious complications, except for the fine hair growing on her face. By then she'd developed dense bilateral cataracts with "hand movement" vision, meaning that she couldn't even see my fingers at four feet, only my moving hand.

It was clear that she needed her cataracts removed. In the meantime, she still required multiple eye drops and a small systemic maintenance dose of prednisone to keep her disease from flaring up. I was able to discontinue the cyclosporine. At that point, she was comfortable and no longer had the severe headaches and eye pain.

As her situation was complicated, I decided to send her to the Uveitis Clinic at the University of California San Francisco Medical Center, where I'd done my fellowship in retina surgery years ago. Their recommendation was to remove the cataracts, but without intraocular lenses. In the 1980s, the general consensus was that IOLs would only make the inflammation worse, probably because of the poorer quality of IOLs at the time, and also perhaps because we had less experience with implantation then.

Having her cataracts removed without putting in the IOLs would require Elena to use contact lenses or thick glasses after surgery, both of which would make it incredibly difficult to work in the fields because of the very hot, dusty conditions in the summer. She would most likely need to continue eye drops, which would be impossible to do with contact lenses, as steroid eye drops consist of a milky suspension that would adhere to the lenses and cloud them up.

I pondered the problem for a few days and asked myself what I would do if I were in her place. I also recalled my own father's struggles with his contact lenses, which he started using after his cataract surgery. He had a history of mild uveitis and was easily treated with prednisone drops. But his ophthalmologist in San Francisco decided against IOLs because he feared they would exacerbate his uveitis.

I decided that, if it were me, the IOLs would be the only practical option, even with the risks. If the inflammation got too severe, the IOLs could be removed later.

When Elena returned the following week, I discussed all the options with her and her mother. She was intelligent and understood the pros and cons of each option. She agreed with my suggestion, and her cataracts were removed and IOLs were implanted, two weeks apart, without incident. In the end, her vision was 20/30 in each eye, and the symptoms of VKH disease never bothered her again.

To this day, Elena continues to do well.

The easy decision for me would have been to follow the recommendation of the Uveitis Clinic at UCSF to simply take out her cataracts and not put in the IOLs. But I'm glad that I stuck my neck out for Elena and recommended them. After 30 years, she never forgot me. Even after I retired to Hawaii, I still get a card from her each Christmas with a photo of her family and a handwritten letter thanking me for being so kind to her, and for putting so much thought into finding the best course of treatment for her.

While I've gotten many cards from patients in the past, Elena is the only one to do so for such a long period. And, while I was still in practice, she would regularly drop off a box of fresh fruit for the office.

If Elena didn't have the IOLs implanted, her life would probably have been much more difficult, and it would have been impossible for her to work in the fields. It always makes me feel good thinking about how I made a difference in her life.

Chapter 22

The Intractable Headache

A FEW WEEKS AGO, I returned to Fresno and had dinner with some of our very old friends from St. Paul Newman Center. In the 1980s, we were all starting out, our children were young and we were all working hard.

Betty Fong became one of my unforgettable patients during that time, even though technically she wasn't really my patient. Looking back at something that happened almost 40 years ago, I was even skeptical if my memories were correct. But Betty was at the dinner to validate those memories.

In the mid-1980s, Betty's husband Roger had decided to quit Valley Medical Center (VMC) and strike out on his own. One of his friends from pharmacy school had bought into a franchise called Medicine Shoppe. It was like a McDonald's franchise, where the company would help the pharmacist purchase drug supplies at the best wholesale price, help with the promotion and running of the pharmacy, and in return a percentage of the profit would be paid back to the company.

We'd known the Fongs since the days of my internship at VMC, and we also attended the same church next to Fresno State University, St. Paul Newman Center, for many years.

Running a small business was a tremendous amount of work and there were risks as well. Both Betty and Roger worked very hard. In addition to being the bookkeeper and all-purpose helper at the pharmacy, Betty also took care of the kids, cooked and did housework.

The Fongs were third- or fourth-generation Chinese. Roger's great-grandfather left China for California to work on the railway, then settled in the Fresno area. The family prospered and owned a large store called the Peacock in southwest Fresno. Roger's grandmother was a devout Catholic and donated a large sum of money to help found the St. Genevieve Church.

Betty's family background was similar. She had grown up in a small foothill town called Lindsey in the San Joaquin Valley. Her family owned a grocery store, which she began working in when she was seven or eight.

We socialized to a certain extent and saw each other on Sundays at church. We noticed when she wasn't there for a few weeks in a row, and learned that she was having a horrible headache that wouldn't go away.

***

I had some experience with headaches. In fact it was people's headaches that made me quit my family practice residency in 1975 after my internship. A significant number of patients at the clinic complained of headaches, and I felt each time I saw a patient with a headache, my own head would ache as well.

As I was the chief resident in the family practice program, I was the main workhorse for the hospital, seeing as many as sixty clinic patients a day. It didn't allow any time for true management of these patients. We simply did the minimal. Usually we would just renew their prescription of Tylenol with Codeine for their headaches.

One of the causes of persistent headaches is a brain tumor. But with so many patients, there was simply no time to do any meaningful workups. It was before the days of MRIs, and regular X-rays were of little help in detecting brain tumors. I often worried that if one of these headache patients turned out to have a brain tumor, I would surely be sued. It was well known that there were informants at the hospital, and if there were any potential malpractice cases, the informant would alert an attorney and collect a finder's fee.

So, I read up on the different types of headaches and prayed that none of my headache patients would turn out to have a brain tumor.

I read that there were essentially two kinds of headaches. Primary Headaches are headaches that are not due to another cause like a brain tumor, infection or another medical condition.

Those that are due to an underlying condition are called Secondary Headaches. Usually, secondary headaches are ruled out early on by imaging studies and lab tests. So most intractable headaches turn out to be primary headaches.

Personally, I'd had to deal with my own headaches. When I was about 9 years old, I was climbing a tree in my village in Hong Kong, trying to pick guava fruits. I lost my balance and fell into the creek, hitting my head on a rock. My head bled, but I didn't tell my parents and the wound healed over in a matter of a week or so and I thought no more of it.

I'd never taken any aspirin or Tylenol, even in college, because I simply grew up not knowing that pain could be treated. During my second year in college, I began experiencing headaches. It was some sort of neuralgia, a sharp pain, and my scalp felt sensitive. These headaches would occur a couple times a year, sometimes lasting for a few days. Not knowing that I could take something for them, I simply put up with the pain and eventually they would go away.

During my last year in college, I finally sought help for my headaches and was evaluated by the doctor at the student health center. He ordered X-rays, which showed that I had a skull fracture that had left an indentation. He thought my headaches were probably caused by the old injury.

It was then that I began taking Tylenol whenever I had a headache. It lessened their intensity, but seldom made them disappear completely.

When I was doing my ophthalmology residency, I would often moonlight as an ER doctor at a hospital in Visalia. I would usually work 24-hour shifts, and on some holidays like Christmas and New Year when other doctors didn't want to work, I would work two or three days straight. Of course, I was often able to sleep for a few hours during the night or when things were slow, such as during dinnertime when few people showed up at the ER.

I saw a lot of patients with headaches in the ER. Some of them were obvious drug addicts who wanted pain meds, often demanding injections of morphine or Demerol. I would offer these patients an alternative treatment such as a Lidocaine injection to numb the muscles in the scalp, which I'd learned from personal experience helped with my own headaches. But the patients almost invariably turned down my suggestion for the injection.

On a few occasions, I was threatened by patients who demanded opiates when I refused them, and at least once I had to ask hospital security to call the police.

***

I learned that Betty had been in the hospital for over a week undergoing all sorts of tests, including EEG, spinal tap to rule out infection and all sorts of imaging studies to try to find a brain tumor, aneurysm or any lesions that might be causing her headache. In addition to her family doctor, she was evaluated by a neurologist, a pain specialist, a neurosurgeon and even a psychiatrist. None of the tests showed any brain tumor, injuries or arthritis in the neck that could be the cause of her horrendous headache.

When I visited her at the hospital, she was on a continuous morphine drip. In spite of this most powerful painkiller, her headache persisted. She was literally crying because of the pain. Light and noise bothered her tremendously.

According to the neurologist's evaluation, migraine was ruled out because she didn't have a visual aura—seeing dark or color spots, sparkles and other visual hallucinations. In a migraine patient, the pain is caused by spasm of the blood vessels, which causes the headache and the visual part of the brain to see things that aren't there. Cluster headaches and other known causes of headaches were also ruled out.

Betty had gone home once, but was again admitted to the hospital because she couldn't bear the pain and there was nothing that would stop it. After another week, even with the intra-venous drip of morphine and other drugs, her headache persisted. Unable to identify the root cause or stop her pain, her doctors again discharged her home. They had nothing more to offer except strong opiates, which didn't help.

A mutual friend called me one Saturday morning to tell me that Betty was doing poorly, and the priest from St. Paul Newman Center, Father Dennis, was at Betty's home to give her Extreme Unction. In the Catholic Church, Extreme Unction is the anointing of the sick. It's a sacrament given to a Catholic whose life is in danger due to sickness or old age.

So, I took my black bag with a couple vials of local anesthetics, i.e. 2% Lidocaine, and a few syringes and headed to the Fong's. When I arrived at their home, Roger was sitting quietly in the living room. The children were at Roger's parents' house. Father Dennis was in the bedroom, sitting a few feet from Betty. All the curtains were drawn and it was completely dark.

I wasn't sure what I could do. In my own case, injections of as little as half a cc of Lidocaine had often been enough to numb the scalp and stop the headache. Sometimes I had to give myself a second dose of half to one cc.

Betty was lying in her bed quietly, her hands covering her eyes. Father Dennis was watching her in silence. Half an hour earlier, he had given her the Extreme Unction.

I shook Father Denis' hand and greeted him in a whisper. I then went to Betty's bedside. She opened her eyes and thanked me for coming.

I thought about all the tests she'd undergone, evaluated by different specialists, and there was nothing they could do for her. What could I, as an ophthalmologist, do?

At this point, Roger entered the room and I said to him, "I don't know if this is going to help. I've had some success with my own headaches by injecting Lidocaine into the scalp muscles. Sometimes, the anesthetic relaxes the muscles and breaks the cycle of spasm. If you wish, I can try on Betty."

I'd spoken softly so I wouldn't disturb Betty, but obviously she heard me because she cried out, "I'm willing to try anything."

"Of course," agreed Roger. "We're willing to try anything."

Father Dennis remained sitting and didn't comment.

I opened my black bag and got out a vial of 2% Lidocaine and a syringe with a one-inch 30-gauge needle. I withdrew about 2 cc of the local anesthetic into the syringe, then took out a few alcohol wipes and cleaned Betty's head at the base of her skull and another spot on top of her head.

I first injected 1 cc at the base of her skull, and another cc on the top of her head. Setting down the syringe, I began massaging the injection areas to help spread the anesthetic. I stayed close to Betty's bed, waiting to make sure she didn't have any reactions to the Lidocaine. I had a few vials of epinephrine and Benadryl in case she had an allergic reaction.

Ten minutes later, Betty opened her eyes and exclaimed, "My headache is gone!"

Father Dennis stood up and made the sign of the cross over her. Roger remained quiet, probably thinking it was too good to be true.

Betty then sat up in bed. After a few minutes, she stood up and walked slowly and unsteadily—she'd been bedridden for weeks—to the bathroom to wash her face.

"I cannot believe my headache is gone," cried Betty as she emerged from the bathroom, moving her head sideways and up and down, as if to test if this was merely a dream.

I hadn't said much, and had just been observing Betty and thinking. I was surprised that the intra-venous morphine drip didn't help, but 2 cc of the Lidocaine made the headache go away. I, too, thought it was too good to be true.

Betty was tremendously relieved to be out of pain. She'd been worried that she was doomed to suffer this headache forever. She gave me a hug and thanked me for making her feel like a human being again.

I don't remember exactly what I said, but it might have been something like, "We know God works in mysterious ways."

In the following forty years, Betty never had another such headache. To this day, I'm not certain what was causing it. The most likely culprit was the tremendous stress she was under, working at the pharmacy and taking care of things at home. I suspect the muscles in her scalp were in spasm and the Lidocaine simply broke the cycle. It was probably the case of a tension headache that had spun out of control.

I was very glad that such a simple treatment cured Betty's headache. Even now, as I think about the incident, the story seems too farfetched. But there were three witnesses there that day, and I know it wasn't my imagination.

Perhaps God answered the Fong's prayers, and I was merely the instrument.

Chapter 23
Wong Choi

I COULDN'T EVEN REMEMBER what sort of dog Wong Choi was, but I think someone told me it was some sort of Cocker Spaniel. It was yellow and not very big, weighing about 20 pounds. Her owner named her Wong Choi, meaning *Yellow Fortunate* in Chinese.

This story is remotely tied to Roger Fong, Betty's husband, although only very tangentially. A new priest from Hong Kong had arrived for the St. Genevieve Church in West Fresno, the church Roger Fong's paternal grandmother had donated money to help build in 1938. It was through the church that I met the priest, and through the priest that I met Wong Choi and her owners.

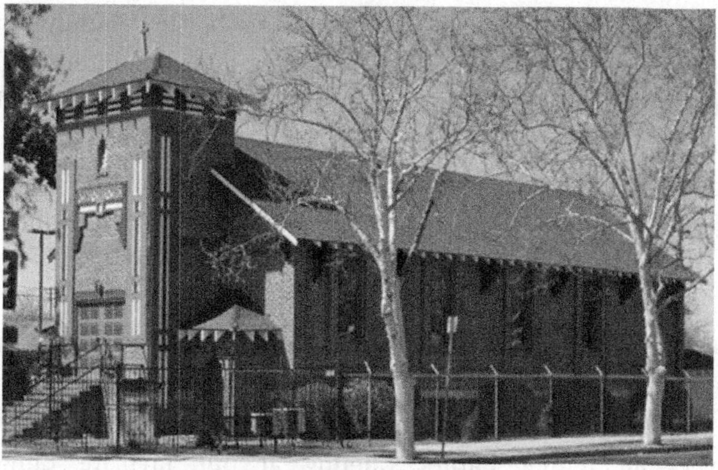

St. Genevieve, Fresno.

I didn't grow up with dogs, so I can't say that I love them. The truth is that I feared them, because when I was about nine years old I was bitten on my right shoulder by a German shepherd, and for several weeks I watched the dog for any foaming at the mouth or bizarre behavior, which I'd learned were signs of rabies. I didn't tell my parents because they were never home. I was petrified that I was going to get rabies, as dogs did carry the virus in Hong Kong in those days. Obviously I didn't get it, but the fear of dogs stayed with me.

The church we attended, the St. Paul Newman Center, was located in northeast Fresno. The St. Genevieve Church was in southwest Fresno, the part of Fresno that most people now avoided. The original purpose of this church was to serve the small Chinese community.

In the early 1900s, the busiest part of Fresno was in the south. Most of the Chinese lived in the area and owned small businesses or restaurants; but much of the next generation got educated, becoming doctors, dentists, pharmacists, teachers and accountants, and as the town grew and spread north, they too moved north.

Roger grew up not far from the church. Their family store, the Peacock, sold clothes, shoes and most household items. After getting his pharmacy degree from UCSF, Roger got a job at VMC and the family moved to the north end of town. So although his grandmother was involved with St. Genevieve's and he grew up attending church there, it made more sense for him and his family to attend the St. Paul Newman Center Church.

After mass one autumn Sunday, Roger told me that he wanted me to meet someone from Hong Kong, a Father Francis Cheung, who was now the parish priest at St. Genevieve's.

I readily agreed, and on a Saturday evening, Roger, Betty, Mary and I met Father Cheung at our favorite Chinese restaurant, the *Imperial Garden*.

Father Cheung was a compact man, less than five feet tall, with a full head of jet-black hair that he wore combed back. He looked younger than his sixty years of age.

"How are you adjusting to Fresno?" I asked.

"So far it's nice," he replied. "It's autumn and the weather is cool. Everyone tells me that it gets really hot in the summer."

"Yes, it does get hot. But it's a dry heat," I remarked with a smile, thinking that he'd find out how hot it could get soon enough.

As we conversed, I found out that Father Cheung was Hakka Chinese like me, but he was from a different area than my parents. He came from an area between the Hakka and Teochew people in northeast Guangdong province; thus he was able to speak both the Hakka and Teochew dialects fluently.

The Toechew people are also called Tie-Chiu in Romanized text, Toechew and Chaozhou in Mandarin, and ChiuChau in Cantonese.

"Oh yes, I know your area," I exclaimed. "We know a Father Joseph Pang from Malaysia, and he was also from there."

Father Pang was the nice priest in Muar, Malaysia who talked my parents into getting baptized as Catholics so that when we had to return to Hong Kong in 1962, they would have an easier time finding teaching jobs in the numerous Catholic schools there. I think Father Pang saved our family. He was correct, because with their baptismal certificates, they both found teaching jobs at Catholic schools.

I related the incident to Father Cheung, and he laughed out loud and exclaimed, "Yes, I know many Chinese rice bowl Catholics!"

When I heard the term, I laughed loudly as well—it was the first time I'd heard the expression, and it certainly described my parents. (Rice bowl Catholics are those who convert for economic reasons.)

"Of course I know Father Pang," he added. "What a small world! Father Pang and I are kind of related. He is now in Mauritius tending to the Chinese Catholics on the island.

"Like him, I just wanted to get out of Hong Kong, to be as far away from the communists as I can," Father Cheung continued.

When the waiter came to take our order, we let Roger, being a food lover, decide what we were having. He ordered a steamed grouper, Chinese deep fried whole chicken, beef and broccoli, fish maw soup and a plate of yellow egg noodles with tiger prawns.

That was how my friendship with Father Cheung began. As the parish got smaller and smaller, the church's finances were getting more precarious. Some months, he wasn't able to pay the high utility bill.

I was at the peak of my career, doing many surgeries and making good money, and I felt good that I was able to support his church as well.

One of the biggest supporters of St. Genevieve's was Mrs. Rosalia Chen. She and her husband had emigrated from Hong Kong some twenty years ago, and now owned a grocery store in a small town in the San Joaquin Valley called Tranquility, about 40 miles from Fresno. The couple had worked very hard, from dawn till midnight, seven days a week, for many years. Now they were financially secure and had bought a house in southeast Fresno, in an area called Sunnyside. They had two children and a dog. Their son, the eldest, was away at college and their daughter, who was about eighteen, lived at home because she had some sort of mental issues and couldn't live independently.

Rosalia Chen prayed daily for her daughter and often made special donations on her behalf, hoping that with her devotion, God would make her daughter's mental issues go away.

Her husband, on the other hand, often complained that she was giving the church too much money, which they had worked so hard for all those years. But he was a nice, quiet man, and he never stopped her from making her donations.

Whenever I had patients at Fresno Community Hospital in the south end of town, I often stopped by St. Genevieve's church and visited with Father Cheung, sometimes going out to lunch at the nearby Far East Café, owned by an old Chinese couple.

One day I received a call from him asking to meet with me. We set up a time, and one Saturday after seeing my patients at the hospital, I met Father Cheung at the Far East Café.

"Dr. Hung, do you remember Rosalia Chen?" Father Cheung asked.

I had met and talked with her at numerous St. Genevieve's church functions, and we had dinner on a couple occasions.

"Of course I do," I replied.

"She would like to ask a big favor of you," he continued.

I smiled and asked, "What sort of a favor?"

"Their dog, Wong Choi, is getting old. It keeps falling into their swimming pool. Finally, they took her to the vet, and Rosalia was told that Wong Choi has very dense cataracts in both eyes and is essentially blind. She asked me if you could remove the cataracts for her dog," he explained.

I was surprised by the request and was silent for a minute. Finally, I said, "Father Cheung, you know I've done many free surgeries for patients who had no insurance and those who couldn't afford to pay. I don't mind doing surgeries on people, but I've never done cataract surgery on a dog."

"Rosalia said if you could do surgery on people, the surgery on a dog should be easier," Father Cheung remarked.

Before I began my ophthalmology residency many years ago, I took a basic science course for ophthalmology at Stanford University and made friends with a veterinarian from the UC Davis Veterinary School, one of the top vet schools in the world. He said he was doing cataract surgeries on dogs, and I learned that, indeed, the school had a veterinarian who specialized in such procedures.

"There's a vet at the vet school at UC Davis who would be happy to take care of Wong Choi," I replied. "First of all, I've never done cataract surgery on a dog. Secondly, I don't even know where I could do it—outpatient clinics or hospitals certainly wouldn't allow it. Another problem is that the dog has to be asleep. So, there are many issues," I explained.

"Dr. Hung, I know it's an imposition," Father Cheung said. "I know you're a very busy man. Rosalia said her husband has to run the store, and she wouldn't know how to get to the UC Davis vet school. I think she has decided that you're the one who should do it."

I'd never liked pushy people. How could Rosalia decide that I should do her this favor? I was a little annoyed.

All my life, when I decided to help people, I often weighed how much effort I had to put out versus how much benefit the other person would get. In this case, Rosalia was asking me to do it for her convenience, and it would be a major effort on my part. In fact, it would take a lot more time for me to do the surgery on a dog than on a person because it wasn't what I did regularly and things weren't set up for me. It would probably take me an entire day to do the procedure, because I would have to arrange to have everything set up beforehand. I was certain that if she really tried, she could find or hire someone to take her to UC Davis, where a qualified vet with the proper set-up could do the job.

Father Cheung was quiet and looked disappointed. I felt bad, as I really liked him. Finally, sounding sad and a little desperate, he said, "Dr. Hung, it would mean so much to me if you would help Rosalia. She's the biggest supporter of the church. I really hate to disappoint her."

"Father Cheung, please let me think it over," I said. "I'll give you a call."

After lunch, as I drove home, I thought about Father Cheung and Father Pang. I considered that sometimes in life we had to do things we didn't want to do. Perhaps this was one of them. Father Cheung probably didn't want to be begging me to help his most generous donor any more than I didn't want to take on the task.

At dinner, I announced to Mary and the children what had transpired at lunch with Father Cheung. They all burst out laughing.

"I hope you won't be arrested for practicing veterinarian medicine without a license," quipped Melissa, our oldest.

Over the next week, my stand softened. I did some reading about cataract surgery for dogs and found out that, at least in the 1980s, they weren't putting intraocular lenses in animals following surgery. Since domestic animals were fed and didn't have to hunt for their food, super sharp vision wasn't required.

At dinner a few days later, I announced that I was seriously thinking about doing the surgery, and explained that dogs didn't need intraocular lenses.

"I know why you don't need to put an intraocular lens in the dog," our ten-year-old son James said. "Because it doesn't read."

We all laughed.

The next day, I called Father Cheung and asked him to get Rosalia to see if her vet would do the anesthesia and if we could do the surgery in his clinic.

The day after that, Father Cheung called to say that Rosalia wanted to meet with me so I could examine Wong Choi.

We met at St. Genevieve's on a Saturday afternoon. Rosalia and her daughter Fiona were there with Wong Choi. The dog was quiet and well behaved as I shone my small flashlight into her eyes, seeing her obvious cataracts. They were chalk-white, meaning that they were very mature. If they weren't removed, the contents of the cataract could leak into Wong Choi's eye and cause severe inflammation, which could lead to irreversible blindness.

I patted Wong Choi on her head, stroking her soft yellow fur. She wagged her tail. It was probably the first time in my life I actually patted a dog.

Rosalia said her vet had agreed to do the anesthesia and would also like to help me with the surgery.

Another ophthalmologist in town, Dr. Zuckerman, caught wind of what I was up to and volunteered to help, saying that he'd helped remove a dog's cataracts while in residency at Yale. It was the ophthalmology department chairman's dog. I was pleased that another ophthalmologist would be helping.

I made a list of instruments needed for the surgery, plus all the medicine and eye drops I would need, and other supplies such as sutures. I was used to doing cataract surgery with an operating microscope, but in this case I'd have to do it with a head-mounted surgery loop (magnifying glasses). A year earlier, I'd bought the best surgery loop made by Zeiss at our annual eye meeting. This one had its own light source. I'd used it for micro-surgeries such as removal of pterygium, and it would work well for Wong Choi's cataract removal.

On a Friday afternoon, with the vet's clinic closed, we prepared for the surgery. As I was unloading all my equipment, including the cryo machine and two heavy tanks of CO_2 gas (which made the cryo machine very cold), I laughed and shook my head. I couldn't believe I'd been suckered into doing surgery on a dog.

The vet, Dr. Odom, was an older man with a full head of white hair and a kind face. He started an IV in Wong Choi's leg and gave her a push of ketamine. Soon Wong Choi was limp and unconscious.

We tried to adhere to human cataract surgery procedures as much as possible. I sterilized the dog's right eyelid and the adjacent area with Betadine solution, and irrigated the cornea and conjunctiva with Neosporin eye drops to prevent infection.

The eye was kept open with a wire speculum. Dr. Zuckerman had also brought his own operating loop. A ceiling-mounted operating light was focused on Wong Choi's right eye. With a sharp diamond blade, I made a small incision at the limbus, the area between the clear cornea and the white sclera. The wound was then enlarged with a pair of small scissors.

Prior to the start of the surgery, I'd tested the cryo machine to make sure it worked. Now, I gently touched the opaque lens with the tip of the probe, and activated the machine with my foot. Ice began to form until the entire lens was an ice ball. In the meantime, Dr. Zuckerman continuously irrigated the cornea with saline solution to keep it from drying. I gently rocked back and forth, and soon the lens was loosened and removed from the eye. I then closed the wound with very thin black nylon sutures, burying the knots in the sclera so they wouldn't cause any irritation.

The surgery on the right eye had gone well, without any complications.

We then turned out attention to the left eye and did the same. It also went well. We applied an antibiotic ointment to both of Wong Choi's eyes but didn't put any eye patches on as we usually did, because it was impossible to keep them taped to the dog's fur.

"We are finished," I declared with a sigh of relief.

Dr. Odom had remained in the background, observing quietly with amazement. "It's fascinating," he exclaimed, as he injected something into Wong Choi's IV. Not long after, the dog began to move a little and slowly woke up.

As Dr. Odom's assistant at the clinic was washing my instruments, Dr. Odom asked, "Dr. Hung, would you do this again if I have a dog that needs cataract surgery?"

I smiled and replied, "Dr. Odom, this was my first and last cataract surgery on a dog. The vet at UC Davis would do a better job because they're geared for such a surgery. Here, we have to make do with so many things. It's just too difficult and too inconvenient. I did it as a favor to Father Cheung and I won't do it again."

Dr. Odom smiled and said, "I totally understand."

Two weeks later, Rosalia invited Mary and me to a dinner at the Imperial Garden. Father Cheung was in a jubilant mood.

"Wong Choi is doing really well," he announced. "She no longer falls into the swimming pool."

As the owner of the restaurant was a good friend of Rosalia's, Wong Choi was allowed to come into the restaurant. I shone my flashlight in her eyes and saw that the surgery had nicely healed and she was looking at me, wagging her tail.

Wong Choi has remained one of my most unforgettable patients. Looking back, I'm glad that I did it and now I have an interesting story to tell, even though at the time I thought it was such an imposition.

More than anything, I was glad that I didn't hear from the California Veterinary Medical Board!

Chapter 24

The Blind People of Southeast Asia

SAIGON FELL TO THE NORTH VIETNAMESE on April 30, 1975. In November of that same year, the first Hmong refugees arrived in the United States.

Initially most of them were settled in Minnesota and Wisconsin because of the churches that had sponsored them. Some Hmong families were sponsored by church groups in Fresno, and later many other refugees began arriving in the Fresno area because they couldn't stand the bitter cold Minnesota and Wisconsin winters.

This first wave was mainly soldiers and workers associated with the US Secret War effort in Laos. They were United States allies in a fight against communist rule, living directly in the conflict zone and in constant danger. The North Vietnamese were hunting the Hmongs down.

The words Hmong and Mong refer to an Asian ethnic group. Their homeland is in China, especially along the Yangtze and Yellow rivers. In the 18th century, Hmong people started moving to other Southeast Asian countries. They never really had a country of their own. Now, they live in many parts of China, northern Vietnam, Laos, Thailand and Myanmar.

Today, the Fresno area has the second-largest Hmong population in the country behind Minneapolis, with about 33,000 people living in the region.

During the last year of my ophthalmology residency, we began seeing Hmong patients who claimed to be blind.

In the US, a person is legally blind if their vision is 20/200 or less in their better eye. That means if an object is 200 feet away and can be seen perfectly by someone with normal vision, a legally blind person would have to stand 20 feet from it in order to see it clearly.

In addition, if a patient's field of vision is less than 20 degrees, i.e. tunnel vision, this would also qualify as legal blindness.

To certify a person as legally blind means that they would qualify for disability benefits for life.

It started with a few, but then we began seeing more and more Hmong patients coming into the clinic for evaluation of their eyesight. These weren't the best kind of patients for a training program, because we usually learned little from them and they took a tremendous amount of time.

In 1977, Dr. Keltner and his colleagues at the University of California at Davis examined 137 patients who complained of vision problems but turned out to have healthy eyes. They were all Laotian (Hmong) refugees. The conclusion by Dr. Keltner and his group was that they were faking it in order to obtain disability payments or awards in lawsuits.

Unlike other specialties like orthopedic surgery, we had some good techniques to rule out false claims. In the case of orthopedic patients complaining of pain, which is subjective, it was often impossible to tell if it was real.

In our training, we were taught to differentiate real blindness, malingering and functional (hysterical or psychosomatic) blindness. True blindness is generally easy to determine, as we can usually find the cause of why the patient can't see—i.e., an issue with the eye itself, the optic nerve or the brain. Malingering can sometimes be difficult to diagnose because of the incentive for these patients to be diagnosed blind. Sometimes this group of patients tries too hard to appear blind, such as frequently running into things or claiming that they can't sign their names. Blind people and people with functional blindness don't usually run into things and can sign their names and even write simple sentences.

I tried to be patient and fair to these patients, but it wasn't easy because I knew most of them were faking it, and it was a waste of our time and resources to examine them.

Many of them were young, between 20 and 50 years old. One patient in her early twenties, a woman named Jia Her, was most trying. She spoke some English but was very slow to answer my questions. It would take her a minute or so to answer a yes or no question, which was a red flag for malingering. It seemed that she was determined to be blind.

I decided to give her one of the simple vision tests called an optokinetic drum—a rotating instrument that the patient sits and faces.

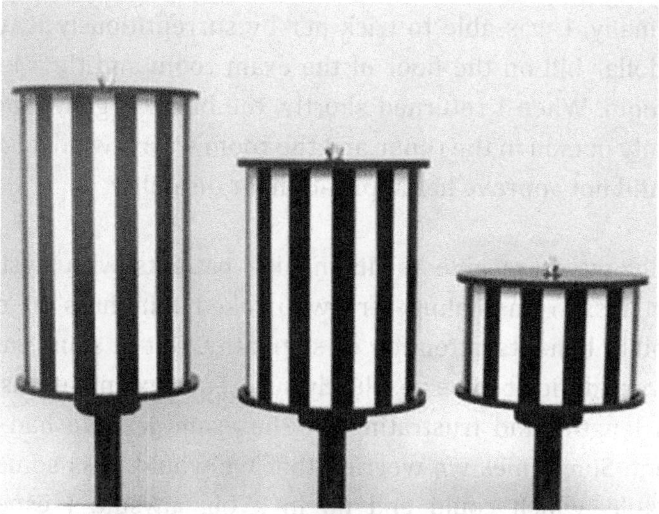

Optokinetic drums of different sizes

Its full name is the optokinetic nystagmus (OKN) drum. The optokinetic reflex allows us to follow objects in motion when the head remains stationary (e.g., observing individual telephone poles on the side of the road as one travels by them in a car). This reflex develops at about 6 months of age.

In the OKN drum test, the patient is asked to look at the spinning drum. The examiner then observes the patient's eye movements carefully. The reflex is involuntary and appears as long as the subject is sighted and is looking at the drum. Some of my patients tried to ignore the drum, but after a while every one of them who was not blind responded to the test.

It didn't measure the acuity of the patient's sight, but showed that their vision was at least 20/200.

I usually scheduled these patients at the end of the clinic day so I'd have extra time if I needed it. Such an examination was often a test of will, an endurance test.

Jia initially tried to ignore the drum; but after half an hour, I noted her eyes tracking the drum back and forth. Of course, she had no idea what I was testing.

Finally, I was able to trick her by surreptitiously leaving a five-dollar bill on the floor of the exam room and then leaving the room. When I returned shortly, the bill was gone. She was the only person in the room, and the room wasn't well lit.

I did not approve her application for disability.

Usually we were able to distinguish patients with hysterical vision loss from malingerers who faked blindness to obtain disability benefits, attention or sympathy. But in some cases, it was very difficult to be absolutely sure. Such examinations were often lengthy and frustrating for the examiner. We had to be patient. Sometimes we worried that we would miss something treatable, which could end up in a big lawsuit. I especially worried when these patients also complained of headaches. In our practice, if a patient complained of headaches and loss of vision, we needed to rule out a brain tumor. Some of them had to have brain scans.

In some cases, when I really couldn't be sure, I would send patients to undergo a sophisticated test known as the VEP (Visually Evoked Response Potential), which measures the electrical response of the brain's primary visual cortex to a visual stimulus with a bright flashing light. These tests are time-consuming and expensive, but if a person indeed cannot see or sees poorly, it would show up in the VEP.

Sometimes, a patient's psyche takes over, producing the conviction that their sight is limited, even when it isn't.

For some children, vision problems can at least partly be explained by psychosocial problems related to divorce, poor academic performance or other critical needs for attention.

One teenage Hmong girl I remember well came in claiming to be unable to see out of one eye. However, when I examined her, I couldn't find anything wrong with her and I was certain that she could indeed see out of that eye. By that point, there was enormous reluctance on her part to admit that she could see.

I told her parents that I'd seen these kinds of things again and again and reassured them that her vision would come back.

It turned out that she was having problems in school. I learned that two weeks later, they went to a Hmong shaman and the girl seemed to go into a trance-like state. Then suddenly, she was able to see again.

One of the Hmong refugees whose application for disability I approved was a sixty-odd-year-old ex-soldier. He claimed that he was tortured by the North Vietnamese and witnessed the executions of his fellow soldiers.

When he came into my clinic, the man was almost in a catatonic state, staring at the floor and never making eye contact with me. He looked like a horribly traumatized human being. On his psychiatric evaluation alone, I would have approved his disability application. How could I expect this man, at his age, who had suffered so much, to try to work in a country where he didn't speak the language?

In the mid-1980s, in my private practice in California, I was seeing a number of Cambodian patients, almost all women, who had been referred to me for evaluation because they couldn't see. A few said they were completely blind, not even able to see light. The rest claimed varying degrees of blurry vision.

Before I started seeing these patients, I'd already read in my ophthalmology journals that ophthalmologists in the US were seeing a phenomenon among Cambodian women who complained of not being able to see; and yet after thorough examinations, and sometimes extensive studies, doctors could find nothing wrong with their eyes.

With the above studies in mind, some doctors accused the Cambodian women of malingering because they wanted to collect disability benefits.

We learned that these Cambodian women had seen so much horror that eventually their minds simply refused to take in any more visual information and essentially refused to see. According to Professor Patricia Rozee-Koker of Cal State University Long Beach, who studied vision complaints of the Khmer Rouge regime's refugees, "These women saw things that their minds just could not accept."

Many of the Cambodians also showed signs of severe depression and post-traumatic stress disorder.

The general consensus by expert psychiatrists and ophthalmologists was that the vision problems were triggered by sights of unimaginable horrors they had witnessed in Cambodia, or by trauma endured by Khmer-speaking Cambodian peasants adjusting to life in the US.

For the most part, the patients were not consciously malingering. One patient told me that she saw her five children and husband killed in front of her; shortly after that she lost her vision. Another woman told me that she watched her husband and four children being taken away in 1975. They never returned. She said she cried daily for three years and when she stopped crying, she couldn't see.

Another patient's daughter told me that her mother lost her vision while living under the brutal rule of the Khmer Rouge. She also told me that the Khmer Rouge usually spared the lives of blind people. Perhaps in order not to be killed, some of these people's minds simply switched off the visual cortex part of the brain, becoming "blind" in order to survive.

Rozee-Koker's studies found that those with the worst vision had spent the most time living under the Khmer Rouge, where they often witnessed executions and experienced beatings, starvation, forced labor, humiliations and separation from their families.

Some of them also went through horrendous changes of life as refugees in camps and in the US, not knowing the language and unable to adjust to a culture so different from their own. Experts speculated that many of the 200,000 Cambodian refugees might be more prone to complain of vision trouble because they tended to be uneducated peasants who experienced difficulty adapting to life in a new country. Unable to cope, their minds told them not to see so they didn't have to deal with the harsh realities of life.

Rozee-Koker said the women "sit isolated in their rooms and live over and over the trauma through horrible nightmares and intrusive thoughts," noting that their vision problems are worse when they feel depressed.

Follow-up of some of my patients showed that with time, as their life conditions got better, their vision also improved. Those who had undergone group psychotherapy seemed to get better sooner.

In contrast to some of the Hmong patients, few of the Cambodian patients consciously faked their blindness.

Hysterical blindness is nothing new. It's been reported among shell-shocked soldiers during World War I and II, children of divorced parents and people involved in traffic accidents.

When a human has seen enough suffering, the mind may decide that the person shouldn't see anymore. It's their way of coping.

Chapter 25
Mr. Fu

NOVEMBER 1989 WAS MY FIRST TRIP to Guilin. I was in Hong Kong with our son James, who was nine at the time, for my high school reunion—La Salle College class of 1964's 25th anniversary silver jubilee.

My brother Paul had been promoted to General Manager at the Sheraton Guilin, so I decided to visit him and his new wife, a Chinese woman he had met in Shanghai.

Guilin in 1989 was very different from now. Most people were very poor. When James and I arrived at the Guilin International Airport, it looked like a third-world airport, with a gray wooden building and drab furnishings. Even the immigration area looked spartan. Standing in the line for 20 minutes in the cold, James caught a cold.

This was shortly after the June 4 Tiananmen Square incident, and the hotel was devoid of tourists. The city was like a ghost town, with few domestic and no foreign visitors.

As James and I walked about the city, we saw local people on their bicycles going about their business. The homes along the river were old and rundown. One house attracted our attention with a sign that read *Snakes for Sale*. We looked inside and were startled to see cages of snakes, some under the beds. The house was these people's home as well as their snake farm.

China looked like a very poor country. I wanted to help the people of Guilin, so I asked my brother if he could help me find out how. Paul contacted the People's Hospital Number 2, which had just been renamed Nan Shi Shang Hospital. It was the largest in Guangxi province, containing over 1,000 beds. I was told that it was a hospital for the soldiers, both Chinese and Vietnamese, during the Vietnam War, and it was now a civilian hospital.

I had a meeting with the head of the hospital, Dr. Jia, and also the head of the eye department, a young doctor named Fan Yang, to discuss how I might get involved.

A year after the initial meeting, I returned with several pieces of important equipment, including a laser machine for the treatment of diabetic retinopathy and other retinal conditions. Dr. Yang had pleaded with me to help them get one, as in the entire province of Guangxi, with a population of over 20 million, there wasn't a single working laser. They'd bought one from a Chinese company in Shanghai, but it never really worked because the aiming beam and the actually delivery of the laser spots weren't the same. This meant that you weren't treating the area in the retina you were aiming at. It was too dangerous to use, because if the laser beam hit the macula (the central vision) by mistake, the eye could be rendered instantly to 20/200 vision, legally blind.

Dr. Yang's own mother had to go Guangzhou for laser treatment of her diabetic retinopathy because he was too afraid to use the Chinese-made laser machine.

Following my first visit, I returned once or twice a year, bringing more equipment and supplies such as intraocular lenses, which China was having trouble obtaining because they were so expensive. I found an Indian company that was manufacturing IOLs in the US, and I was able to get them for less than $20 US each, compared to the over $100 the hospital was paying at the time.

In the early 1990s, the salary of a teacher in Guilin was less than $100 US a month, and the salary of the doctors at the hospital was only slightly higher. So $100 US was a great deal of money.

Over the years, I returned to Guilin regularly, bringing equipment, giving lectures and doing surgeries.

In 1998, I took Mary and our three girls, Melissa, MaryAnne and Elizabeth, on a tour of Hong Kong and China for just over three weeks. Elizabeth was still in high school and the older girls were in college. We first visited Hong Kong, then Beijing, Shanghai, Xian to visit the Terra Cotta warriors, and our last destination was Guilin.

While I was doing surgery and seeing patients one day, Mary and the girls were given a tour of the hospital by Dr. Jia. The girls were horrified to see so many very sick patients, some with advanced cancer and brain tumors, burn patients with disfigured faces and children with tubes through their noses. Dr. Jia also took them to an orphanage where the children sang and danced for them.

That evening, Dr. Jia had arranged a banquet in our honor. It was held in the hospital dining room, with about a hundred doctors and nurses present.

The banquet's theme was local cuisine. One of dishes was roast pangolin; another was braised civet cat. Other dishes included deep-fried snake and silken chicken soup with snake meat.

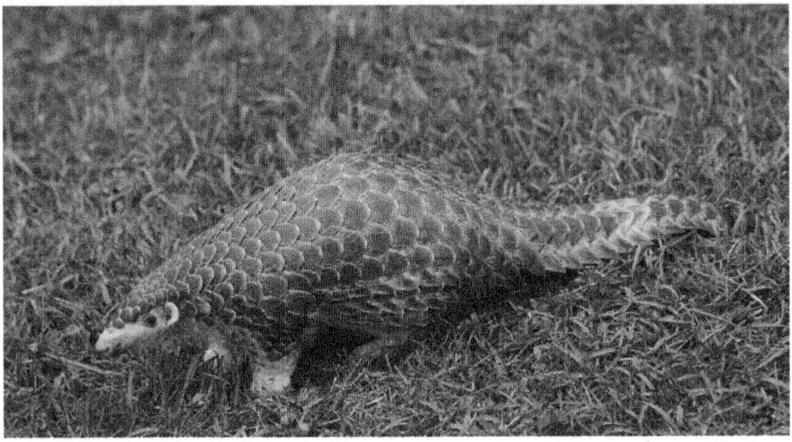

A Chinese Pangolin, sometimes known as a scaly anteater. Some describe it as a Chinese Armadillo (meaning "little armored one" in Spanish).

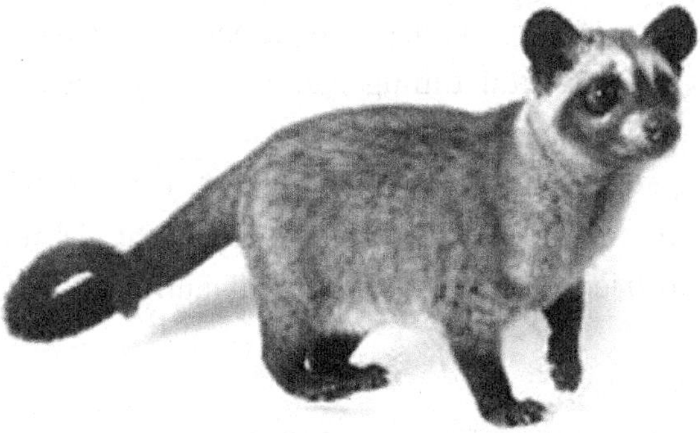

A civet cat is a small, lean, mostly nocturnal mammal native to tropical Asia and Africa, especially the tropical forests.

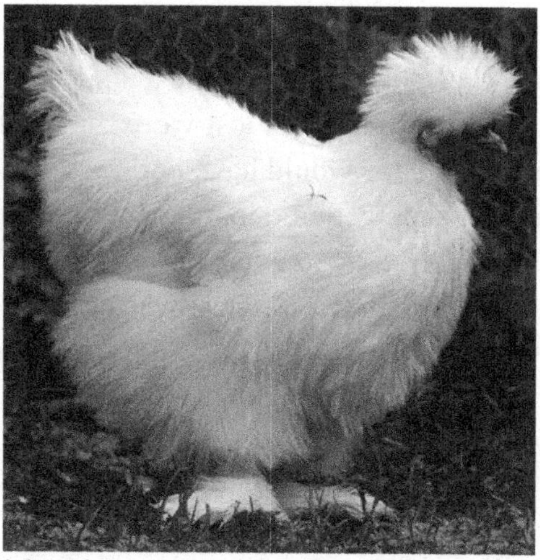

The Silkie (also known as the Silky, Silken or Chinese silk chicken) is a breed of chicken named for its atypically fluffy plumage, which is said to feel like silk or satin. It usually has white feathers and black meat, bone and skin.

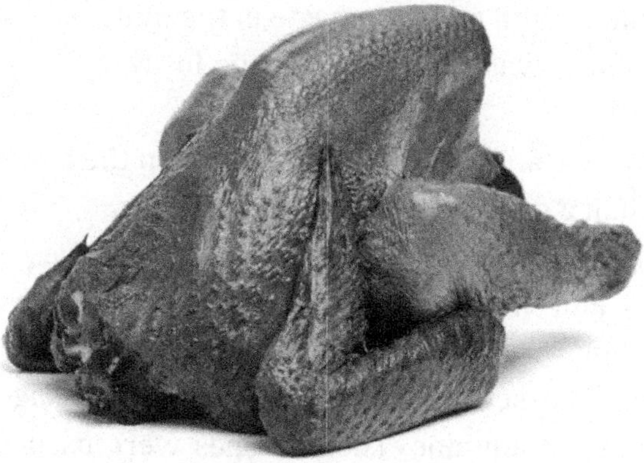

A Silkie chicken's black meat

When the soup was brought to the table, the girls were truly surprised that the chicken's skin, meat and even bones were black. What horrified them the most were the black chicken feet floating in the soup. They would have nothing to do with it.

Dr. Jia, not realizing that most Americans don't even eat organ meat like liver, tried to educate our girls by explaining to them what sort of animal the civic cat was and how the pangolin was similar to the armadillo. The girls' faces turned green. They couldn't understand how people could eat such strange wild animals. Having grown up in a culture that ate almost anything, I had no problem eating any of the dishes.

In the end, the girls didn't go hungry. They liked the duck egg omelet with tomatoes, stir-fried Chinese broccoli and a large, wok-fried sweet and sour fish.

For dessert, they served the local favorite of a dark, gelatinous cake made from a plant root dug up high up in the mountains. I always asked for this dessert whenever I was in Guilin. Our girls wouldn't touch it, but they liked the deep-fried Chinese donuts with red bean paste in the middle.

The banquet was truly an education for them.

On a Sunday, we all went for a boat cruise on the famous Li River and spent half a day in the town of Yangshuo.

Yangshuo is famous for its epic water caves filled with stalagmites and stalactites, underground mud baths, waterfall pools and hot springs. The Longmen Water Cave is the largest underground karst cave, with labyrinthine passages running through three mountains. The passages were used as a refuge during World War II.

As with my previous trips, my visit in to Guilin was mentioned in the newspaper. There were discussions among the readers and hospital employees, and some of them concluded that I must be so rich I didn't need to work, and my children would never have to work for a living either. At the time, philanthropy was unheard-of in China.

There were discussions of my true motives and suspicions that I must have a hidden agenda. Some people simply couldn't understand why someone would donate time and money without getting anything in return!

In spite of China calling itself a communist country, in practice it was far from the truth. The government provided little funds to the hospitals. This was a transitional period in China's economic system, and the hospitals were ordered to operate self-sufficiently. It was difficult to do when most of the patients were very poor. A farmer made much less than $100 a month. If one of their family members got sick, they often had to sell a cow or a few pigs to pay for medical expenses.

One day in the clinic, I saw a man of about sixty, although he looked closer to eighty, with a detached retina. After examining Mr. Fu, Dr. Yang and I agreed that he needed surgery to repair the detachment.

Mr. Fu said he was an unemployed factory manager in a now-closed cement plant. Most of his family and relatives were unemployed as well, because in the 1990s the government was trying to close all the money-losing state industries.

The hospital gave Mr. Fu an estimate of the cost for hospitalization, which was $10 US a day, and he would be in for at least five days. The use of the surgery suite and supplies would be about $200 US. The total cost for him would be about $300 US. By US standards, this was incredibly cheap, but Mr. Fu simply didn't have that kind of money, and he had no cow or pigs he could sell.

In China, if a patient didn't have the required deposit, even a traffic accident victim with critical injuries wouldn't be treated. This was why most Chinese didn't trust doctors, even though it wasn't in fact the doctors who made such decisions. It was the administrators and the government. In order to survive, the hospital had to collect fees from the patients; otherwise, they wouldn't be able to pay the doctors and hundreds of employees needed to keep it running. Doctors were often beaten up, even killed in a few cases, because patients died and their families wanted someone to pay, and it was usually the doctors they came into contact with.

I told Dr. Yang that I would pay the $300 for Mr. Fu's hospital costs, in addition to doing the surgery for him. Mr. Fu was very grateful and bowed deeply to me, at a full ninety degree angle, to express his gratitude.

Dr. Yang assisted me in the surgery, which lasted about one hour. We did the usual scleral buckle, and the retina was reattached without any complications. Mr. Fu was discharged from the hospital as planned five days later.

Mary and I and the girls were staying at the Sheraton Guilin Hotel. We were in our room one day, getting ready to visit the most famous limestone caves in the Guilin area. As we were about to leave, I got a call from the front desk saying someone wanted to see me.

When I went down to the lobby, Mr. Fu was waiting for me. He had brought his wife and son, and had come to thank me. He presented me with a small painting on rice paper of the scenery of the Li River, and also a long letter.

After I said goodbye to the Fu family, I joined Mary and the girls and we got into the van for the limestone cave tour. During the drive, I opened Mr. Fu's letter. It was four pages, single-spaced and in beautiful handwriting.

The letter was written in simplified Chinese writing, so I had to read it slowly, because I'd been educated in traditional Chinese writing in Hong Kong. However, I was able to understand almost everything he'd written.

In the letter, Mr. Fu explained that his real name was Hung, like mine, and not Fu. When he was a baby, he was adopted by a family in the Guilin area. He explained that he had done extensive research on the genealogy of his real family and my own family, and he concluded that we shared the same ancestors, a couple hundred years ago. Since we were relatives, he wanted his family to meet my family.

I sighed and refolded the letter. Having lived in Hong Kong, I'd seen my share of scams. This was an obvious scam.

The following day, as we were getting ready for another outing, Mr. Fu showed up at the reception desk again and insisted on meeting with me. I told the receptionist that I had no desire to meet with Mr. Fu, and that he was not my relative as he was claiming.

Mr. Fu left another long letter. In this one, he pleaded with me to help support his older son, who had just started university in Nanning, the capital of Guangxi province.

I was very annoyed that he was behaving like the fabled camel in the tent. First, I did a free surgery for him, then I paid for all his hospital expenses, and now he wanted me to support his son's college education.

That evening, Mr. Fu again showed up at the hotel and insisted on seeing me. When I told the receptionist that I wouldn't, Mr. Fu said he refused to leave until I met with him.

At that point, hotel security called the police and escorted him away from the hotel.

It's true that desperate people do desperate things. Of course I felt sorry that Mr. Fu was so poor. But I truly owed him nothing.

No, I didn't have so much money that I didn't need to work. I was doing charity work because I felt it was the right thing to do. I worked very hard for my living, and my children would too.

I did feel bad for this man who probably had to struggle all his life. He was a sad sight to behold. He had hollow cheeks, a gray face, thinning gray hair and missing teeth—and those still in his mouth were brown, stained by his years of smoking.

I thought if I were in his situation, I might have done the same thing. By his reasoning, I had so much money that I was able to donate a laser machine worth $45,000 US, so what was a few hundred dollars to me, to help his son?

Should I have given in and helped him? Like beggars in China in those days, if you gave to one, a whole crowd would surround you.

A case in point was our experience in the local marketplace a day earlier. We tried to be fair by buying a dollar or two of fruit from each vendor; but finally, we'd bought more than we could eat, and we stopped buying. There was one hefty woman at the end of the row selling watermelon who we didn't buy from. She began screaming at us for not being fair to her, and launched into a tirade against us. Our girls were startled that this woman could be so abusive simply because we didn't buy from her.

Again, desperate people do desperate things. The culture was very different from that in the US. I speculated that because many of these people's lives were extremely difficult, they felt that people like us owed them something and it was our responsibility to help them.

If I'd agreed to pay for Mr. Fu's son's education, no doubt I would have been faced with more such demands, if not from Mr. Fu then perhaps from others.

Someone once told me that there are countless poor people on this earth, and I can't help all of them. The same person also told me never to let someone else's problem become mine.

I've always tried to the right things in life. I often wonder if I should have helped Mr. Fu with his son's education. He was right that a few hundred dollars a year for several years wouldn't have made a big difference to me. But as humans, I think we like to help people on our own terms. When they get too pushy or we feel we're being taken advantage of, we get upset and perhaps even become a little mean.

Looking back, I wish I had helped. It wouldn't have been much effort on my part, but Mr. Fu's son would have benefitted greatly.

Mr. Fu taught me that life is not black and white. Sometimes we try to make the decision we think is right, but later on, when our own thinking and philosophy changes, we wish we'd done differently.

Chapter 26
The Paintball Injury

BEFORE I RETIRED FROM PRIVATE PRACTICE, I was getting tired of the rat race. There was too much paperwork—so much that it was taking away from time I could be spending with my patients.

The working environment for doctors was getting worse every year. I was fortunate to be in ophthalmology, and I wasn't harassed as much as the primary care doctors were. Some of my friends who had graduated from medical school in the mid-1970s were working over 60 hours a week, almost as hard as when they were interns, just to make ends meet: to pay their rent, nurses and other office expenses on the highly reduced reimbursements they got from HMOs, Medicare and Medicaid. And then a huge part of what was left went to pay for malpractice insurance.

Much of their frustration was more than just the money. It was the intrusion on their autonomy. Many of them spent endless days and long years acquiring an extraordinarily specialized skill, only to find themselves being told by some young administrator, often with little medical training, how many minutes they could spend with a patient, how long they could keep a patient in the hospital and what sort of treatment they were allowed to give.

With the EHR (Electronic Health Records) being made mandatory by the government, many doctors spent countless hours keying information into computers that few people would ever read. A case in point was an appointment I had with my internist, during which she sat in her chair at the desk and only asked questions while keying in my responses. She never once got up to examine me and there was little eye contact because she was busy looking at the computer screen. The human touch of being a medical doctor was gone.

I'd been luckier than most because I truly did enjoy my practice and I quit before the EHR became mandatory. I decided that it was time to do something else, such as writing and doing more charity work in developing countries.

Going on a medical mission is different from working in your own practice because you know you're doing something good, helping people who would otherwise not get the help and making a difference in people's lives.

In 2014, my good friend John Paopao, a Samoan plastic surgeon in Hilo, Hawaii, invited me to go on a medical mission to Samoa, previously known as Western Samoa.

Although I went to share my knowledge and expertise, the two weeks I spent in Apia were educational for me as well. I was grateful for my years of experience and felt I could handle any eye problems we encountered there. Many general ophthalmologists weren't comfortable treating the retina, but since I'd taken a fellowship in retina surgery, I was confident dealing with most eye conditions. The only exceptions would be the repair of a tear duct in an eyelid injury or a fracture of the eye orbit.

One evening, after a busy day at the eye clinic at the General Hospital in Apia, I took one of the colorfully painted local buses, which cost me about fifty cents, back to the Annabelle Inn where all of us on the medical mission were staying.

As we were having dinner in the hotel restaurant, Milly, the slim young Samoan woman from the front desk, came by the table and said someone at the hospital wanted to speak to me. It was Dr. Schultz, the young intern who had been shadowing me in the eye clinic.

"Dr. Hung, I hate to bother you," Dr. Schultz said apologetically, "but I have a patient that I don't know what to do about. Dr. Taloa is helping her husband at his church, and she suggested that I call you to see if you'd be interested in taking care of him." Dr. Taloa was the only ophthalmologist in the country, and her husband was a Lutheran minister in town.

"What sort of problem does the patient have?' I asked.

"It's a fifteen-year-old boy," Dr. Schultz answered. "He and his brother and two other friends were shooting at each other in a war game with their paintball guns. This boy was hit in his right eye with a paintball. I can't see the pupil—I think there's blood inside his eye."

At the time, Dr. Schultz had only spent a couple of months working in the eye clinic with Dr. Taloa, and really knew very little about ophthalmology. I told him I'd like to help and that I would be at the eye clinic in about half an hour.

I returned to the dining table to finish my dinner and announced to the rest of the group that I had to go take care of an eye patient.

By the time I arrived at the clinic in a taxi, it was after 7 pm and already dark. Dr. Schultz was waiting for me at the door, while Sophie, the clinic nurse, waited in the examining room with the patient.

The patient was sitting in a chair with his parents next to him. He looked more like a mature man than a 15-year-old boy, over 6 feet tall and at least 200 lbs. He had a blue plastic eye shield covering the injured right eye. I learned that his name was Fred. He looked scared and had tears in his left eye.

Sophie introduced me to his parents, saying, "This is Dr. Hung, an eye specialist from Hawaii. He is here for two weeks to help us. He's the best."

The parents stood up and shook my hand. They seemed educated and later I learned that the father was a bank manager and the mother a schoolteacher.

"What happened?" I asked.

The father looked embarrassed and said, "It's all my fault. Last year when I went to Honolulu on a business trip, I bought four paintball guns, one for each of my two boys and their cousins. I told them they had to wear goggles when they played war games. Fred took off his goggles to load the paintballs when his cousin accidentally shot him. It looks like it hit his eye and now he can't see."

A paintball gun or paintball marker, is an air gun used in the shooting sport of paintball. Paintball guns use compressed gas, such as carbon dioxide (CO_2) or compressed air, to propel dye-filled gel capsules through the barrel to hit a target.

The term "marker" is derived from its original use as a tool for forestry personnel to mark trees and ranchers to mark wandering cattle. When the gel capsule (paintball) hits the target, it burst and the paint splatters.

"Let's see what sort of damage you have," I said to Fred, as I led him to a chair in front of a slit lamp.

I carefully removed the eye shield. The lids were a little swollen but not shut. With a sterile cotton tip applicator, I lifted Fred's upper eyelid to get a better view of his eye. I couldn't see the pupil and his eye seemed to be filled with blood, as Dr. Schultz had noted. I gently touched the eyeball and it felt soft, which meant there was a wound that was leaking fluid from the eye.

I moved Fred's chair closer to the table and placed his chin in the cup of the slit lamp. Even with the brightest light the lamp could produce, I still wasn't able to see the pupil.

I asked Sophie if the eye clinic had an ultrasound machine. Such a machine would help to assess the extent of the damage, such as the amount of blood or if the retina was detached.

"Sorry, Dr. Hung. The machine broke a few months ago," Sophie replied. "We haven't been able to send it to New Zealand for repair."

"The light is very bright," complained Fred.

"That's a good sign," I remarked, "because it means that the retina is probably alright."

I told Fred's parents that I'd treated a few similar eye injuries. "I'm quite sure that there's a wound at the limbus of the eye," I explained. "The limbus is the area between the cornea, which is the clear part of the eye, and the white of the eye. It's dangerous to try examining it more because we may do more damage. What Fred needs is to be put to sleep so I can carefully examine the extent of the damage and repair it."

"When should it be done?" Fred's father asked.

"As soon as we can, probably tonight," I replied. "We need an anesthesiologist. Sophie will do some calling to see if one is available tonight."

I carefully put the eye shield back, covering Fred's eye. He was quiet and seemed frightened.

Soon Sophie returned and announced that Dr. Wang, a doctor with the Chinese Medical Team, would be available to help us.

The surgery was set up for midnight. We couldn't do it earlier because Fred had eaten a hamburger at about 4 pm, just before the paintball fight. With food in his stomach, putting him under anesthesia might cause him to vomit, which could do severe damage to the lungs.

Dr. Wang arrived just before midnight. She was a petite woman of about forty years old. Her English was limited but I was able to communicate in Mandarin with her, and found out that she was from the Shanghai area. She inserted a needle into a vein in Fred's left wrist and began a drip of normal saline. This was needed because medication could be given to Fred through this intravenous route.

Shortly after, a surgical nurse named Elizabeth arrived and began setting thing up. With Fred on the operating table, the surgical nurse handed Dr. Wang a vial of antibiotics, which I had ordered, for her to infuse into Fred's IV. This would help prevent infection.

Dr. Wang soon put Fred to sleep.

Dr. Schultz was excited that he was able to participate in an eye surgery.

I carefully cleaned the area around the eyelid with Betadine solution. Under the operating microscope, I was able to see a wound from the 1 o'clock to the 3 o'clock area. The area in front of the pupil was filled with blood. With a blunt-tipped irrigating needle and syringe, I gently irrigated BSS (balanced salt solution) into Fred's eye.

BSS is used to maintain the natural condition of the eye during a surgical procedure such as cataract surgery.

Once the blood clot was removed, I was able to see the pupil. It was round, indicating that the iris wasn't damaged. To my relief, the lens behind the pupil was clear and not damaged. If it had been, the surgery would have been more complicated. I would have needed to remove the damaged lens, and then decide if I should replace it with an intraocular lens during the surgery, or wait until later when the wound had healed.

I placed four very fine black silk sutures to close the wound and injected more BSS to re-inflate the eyeball.

With the indirect ophthalmoscope, I was able to examine the retina carefully and was very pleased to see that there appeared to be no damage. If there was blood in the vitreous, it would mean that I wouldn't be able to examine the retina to tell if it was damaged or not. In the US, if there was blood inside the eye, we would use a vitrectomy machine to remove it. But in Apia, there was no such machine. Lucky for Fred, his retina seemed uninjured.

The surgery took a little more than an hour.

I explained to Fred's parents that Fred was very lucky the damage wasn't more severe. Now, we just had to wait to see how it healed, and make sure there were no signs of infection.

A few years earlier, I treated a boy who was also shot in the eye with a paintball gun. The paintball hit right in the center of this poor fellow's left eye and caused the eye to rupture. The damage was extensive. His lens was dislocated into the vitreous and I had to fish it out. He needed many more surgeries after that. The retina was also damaged. Eventually we were able to save his eye, but he only had 20/200 vision.

When I saw Fred initially, I thought he might lose his eye, so I was very pleased with how things eventually turned out.

When accidents like Fred's struck, it always seemed to involve several unforeseen situations. In this case, Fred wasn't wearing his goggles. Usually the socket protects the eye, but the paintball just happened to hit Fred right in the eye. He was very lucky that the paintball probably hit the eye at an angle, and not directly. If so, the damage would have been more severe, as it had been for the other boy.

By the time we finished, it was after 2 am. Fred was admitted to the hospital to continue intravenous antibiotics to prevent infection. His father gave me a ride back to the hotel. He was most grateful that we were able to save Fred's eye. If such an injury went untreated, as happens in some parts of the world, the eye would become infected and be lost.

It was times like those when I was very glad I'd gone into medicine. I did make a difference in Fred's life.

I thanked Fred's father for the ride, and crawled into my bed and soon fell sound asleep, oblivious to the barking feral dogs outside and the intermittent falling mangoes hitting the corrugated tin roof of the Annabelle Inn.

Chapter 27

The Triple Procedure

IN THE MID-1980S, there were fewer retina specialists in the country. In the vast San Joaquin Valley, I was the only solo practitioner. The other two specialists were part of large groups of over ten ophthalmologists, and I was getting most of the referrals from other solo practitioners. As most of the smaller towns in the Valley were served by optometrists instead of ophthalmologists, I was getting most of the referrals from them as well. Many of these optometrists complained that once they referred their patients to the large clinics, they never saw them again. They also complained to me that very often, the ophthalmologists in the large groups said unkind words about the referring optometrists, suggesting that their care was substandard.

Originally inhabited by the Yokuts and Miwok peoples, the San Joaquin Valley is now the backbone of California's modern and highly technological agricultural industry. California ranks as the largest agricultural producing state in the nation. San Joaquin Valley crops include grapes, tomatoes, hay, sugar beets, nuts, cotton and a multitude of other fruits and vegetables.

Although the Valley is predominantly rural, it does contain urban centers such as Fresno, Bakersfield, Stockton, Modesto, Tulare, Visalia and Merced. Fresno is the largest city within the region and the fifth largest city in the state, with a population of over one million.

There are numerous small towns spread throughout the Valley. Many of my patients were from these remote towns, some having to drive for hours to reach my office. Some of them lived up in the mountains.

Realizing their hardship, I often tried my best to provide as complete a care as I could so they didn't have to make extra trips to my office.

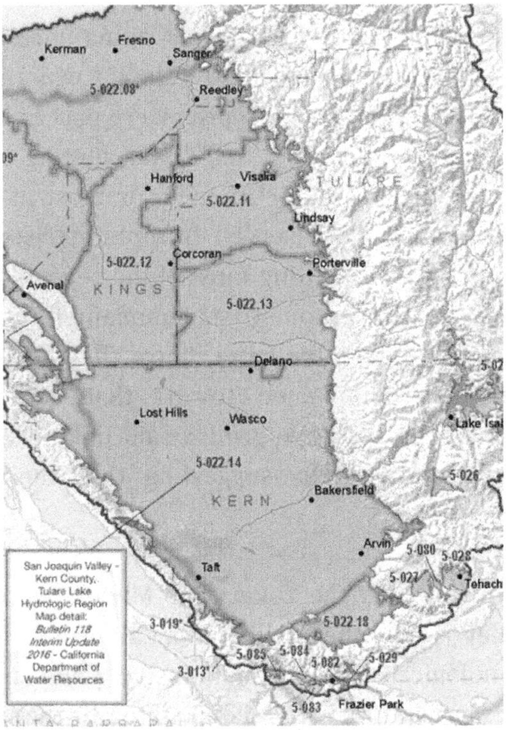

San Joaquin Valley

Harold Hold was a tall, distinguished 70-year-old man who was referred to me because of bleeding in his eye as well as cataracts. He'd had diabetes since he was in his twenties.

He was a retired professor of music at the Fresno State University and used to be the main cello player in the New York Philharmonic Orchestra when he was attending the Juilliard

School of Music. Later, he also played in the Fresno Philharmonic. After his retirement, he and his wife (whom he met at Julliard and who happened to be part Hawaiian) moved up to the mountains so they could enjoy nature. A few years earlier his wife had died, and now he lived alone.

An examination of Harold's eyes showed dense cataracts in both eyes. In the right eye, there was dense vitreous hemorrhage, which he claimed had happened over a year ago. His left eye also showed dense cataract, but I was still able to examine the retina. The retina in his left eye showed new blood vessels in multiple areas. It needed laser treatment to prevent it from hemorrhaging as it had in the right eye.

The vision in Harold's right eye was only light perception, and his left was 20/200. Because he lived alone, and used to read a great deal, it was imperative to help Harold get his vision back as swiftly as possible.

I sat down with Harold and his niece, a forty-year-old schoolteacher who had driven him to my office. They both lived up in the mountain near the entrance to Yosemite National Park. In the winter, the drive could be very difficult as it was often covered with snow.

I explained to them that Harold's left eye—the good eye—needed laser treatment, which I could do that day in the office during my lunch break, after I'd caught up with seeing the other patients.

The treatment plan for the right eye would be cataract surgery, followed by vitrectomy to remove the blood. Once I could see the retina, then I would treat it with laser to prevent further hemorrhage. If everything went well, I could also put an IOL in that eye. In summary, I would be doing four procedures in one sitting.

I'd searched the literature and couldn't find any previous reports of such a surgery. In those days, a person with Harold's problems would usually have the vitrectomy done by a retina specialist, and also have his retina treated with laser. Then the retina specialist would refer him to another doctor for the IOL implantation. It would involve many visits. Living up in the mountain, and now unable to drive, each visit would be a major effort for Harold.

He and his niece were pleased that I was trying to make things easier for them.

At noon, I treated Harold's left eye with extensive laser photocoagulation.

Two weeks later, Harold was admitted to the hospital for the surgery on his right eye. The cataract was so dense that I couldn't see inside the vitreous cavity, which was full of blood. The first step of the surgery was to remove the cataract, which was done successfully. Then I did the vitrectomy and cleared the old blood. Visualization of the retina showed multiple areas of neovascularization, so I treated that eye with laser photocoagulation to prevent any further hemorrhage.

When I saw that everything had gone very well, I placed the IOL, which also went very well.

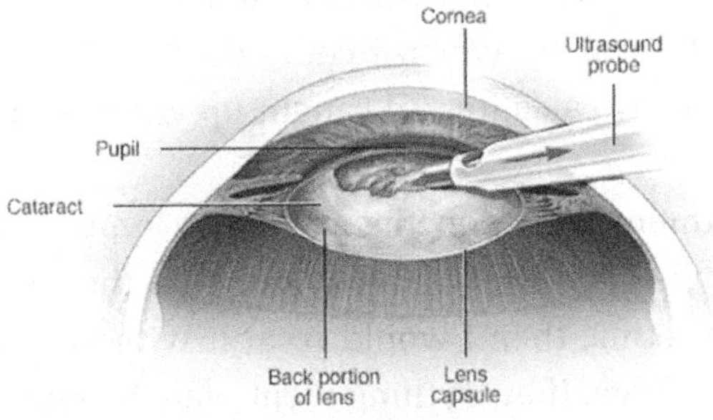

Removing a dense cataract

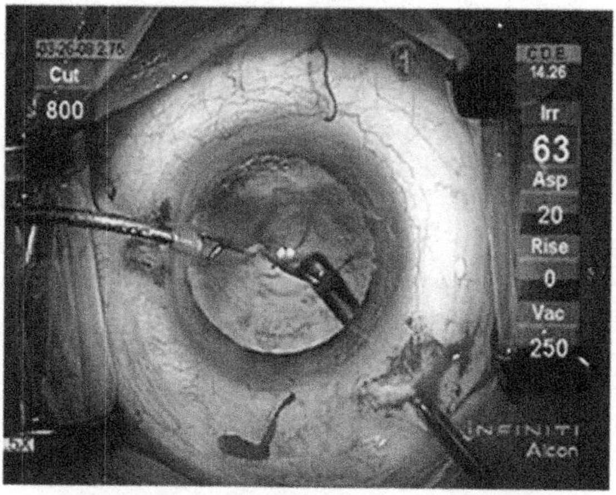

Removing the rest of the cataract

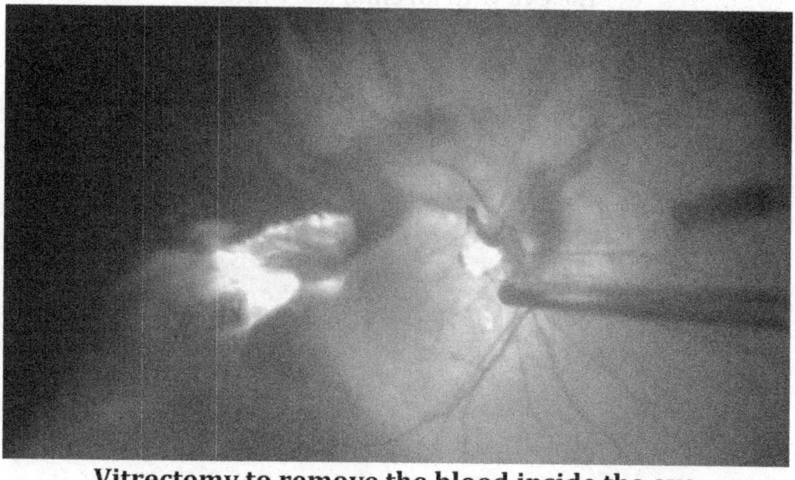

Vitrectomy to remove the blood inside the eye

Instruments include a light pipe, a suction cutter and micro forceps.

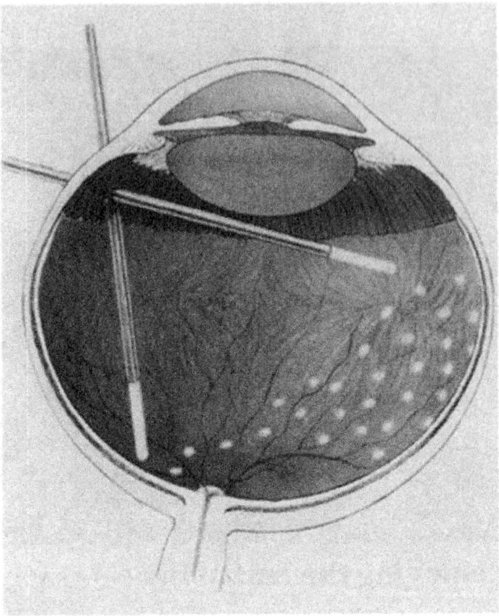

After the vitrectomy, I had a good view of the retina. Laser treatment (endo laser photocoagulation) was done inside the eye with an endo laser probe.

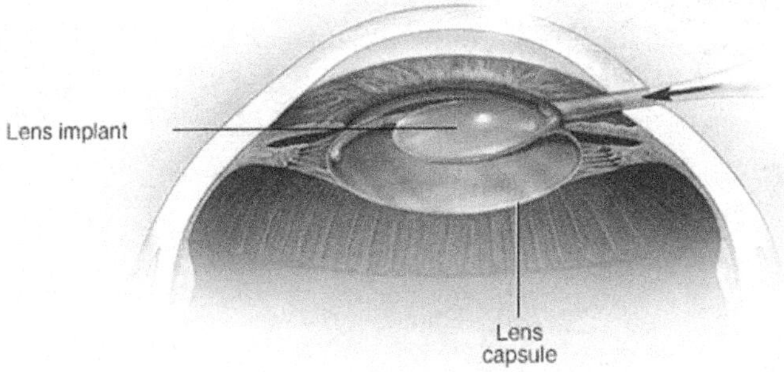

The last step: placement of the IOL

Dr. Bob Mendoza, who was my assistant surgeon, was amazed to see what I was doing. He said he'd never seen this sort of surgery all done in one sitting and suggested that I should write up the case for publication.

Harold did very well post-operatively. The vision in his right eye was now 20/30. The cataract in his left eye was removed a month later, and that also went well. The left eye, too, turned out to have 20/30 vision. He was able to read and drive again.

A few weeks later, another similar patient was referred to me. She was a woman in her sixties who also had a long history of diabetes. She lived in Porterville, a town in the foothills, a difficult drive of two to three hours to the office. Again, I proposed the same treatment plan.

The surgeries went well. Both patients were extremely pleased with the results and were grateful that I was able to do everything in one sitting.

I wrote the two cases up and the article was published in *Annals of Ophthalmology* as the first cases of Triple Procedure Plus—i.e., (1) Cataract extraction, (2) Vitrectomy, (3) Intraocular lens placement, plus (4) Endo-laser photocoagulation.

Perhaps it should have been named the Quadruple Procedure! However, the laser photocoagulation might not have been considered a true surgical procedure.

This was a seminal paper regarding such surgeries. Following publication of that paper, I later came across a few articles describing similar surgeries and they had cited my paper.

It seemed ridiculous that, for an organ as small as the eye, surgeons further sub-specialized into just the cornea, the retina, glaucoma, or just cataract. Because eye surgery is very unforgiving and the learning curve is usually steep, most ophthalmologists would only do surgery they were very good at and comfortable with.

Few general ophthalmologists would attempt a vitrectomy surgery because it's such a delicate surgery in which we actually put instruments inside the eye. On the other hand, few retina specialists would do IOL implants in those days. In my case, I had a fellowship in retina surgery and vitreous surgery so I was comfortable with both. In my residency, I had also mastered cataract surgery and IOL implantation, so I saw no reason why I couldn't do all those procedures for a patient in one sitting.

Again, eye surgery is extremely unforgiving, and the first chance is usually the best chance of a successful surgery.

Being a surgeon means solving your patient's problem as best as you can. It's easy just to do what's always been done and not try new things. But new methods were invented because some surgeon decided to try something different or find a better way to do things.

To me, each surgery is a challenge and it always feels good to meet that challenge. A philosopher once said, "The last thing you want is to have your life become a routine." I totally agree with that. Challenges make one's life exciting.

Chapter 28
Mrs. Lucy Hamilton

MRS. LUCY HAMILTON WAS A CLASSY LADY. She belonged to the older generation of women who always dressed beautifully. Her caramel-colored hair was always perfectly coiffured, and her face was always powdered.

She was always friendly and appropriate. Through our conversations, I learned that one of her sons lived in Paris, and was the head of American Express in France, and Mrs. Hamilton had lived there for a time. Another one of her sons was a cardiologist in Portland, Oregon. She lived with her younger daughter, who was married to a prominent lawyer in town. I never felt that she was telling me how important her family was to impress me. She was just a very nice woman. She told me that I reminded her of her son, the doctor.

She was referred to me because her cataracts were growing and beginning to bother her while driving, especially at night.

I reviewed the possible risks and complications with her and her daughter Marsha, specifically the possibility of infection, which was very rare, in the vicinity of 1 in 1,000. Fortunately, of the many cataract surgeries I'd done, none of my patients had come down with an infection. But when it happened, it could be very serious.

As her cataracts were interfering with her life, Mrs. Hamilton decided to go ahead with the surgery on her right eye first.

She was almost a perfect candidate for cataract surgery, as her eyes were large and rested in the socket in such a way that was easy to access during surgery. Surgery on deep-set eyes was more difficult, because it was like working in a hole. Mrs. Hamilton's cataracts, at 20/80, were just the perfect stage to use phaco (ultrasound) as they weren't too hard. Her skin was always clean, which lessened the chance of germs getting from the skin into her eyes during surgery. She was also a calm person, which made the surgery itself less stressful for the surgeon.

Every step of the surgery went perfectly well from removing the cataract, to cleaning up and implantation of the IOL. It lasted just over twenty minutes. It was also recorded, as I was recording all of my surgeries by then.

The following morning, a Friday, Mrs. Hamilton came in for follow-up.

"How are you feeling?" I asked.

"There's a dull ache in my eye and it's sensitive to light," she responded.

I had her sit in front of the slit lamp so I could examine the eye. What I saw startled me. There was a layer of yellowish-white sediment consisting of pus (i.e., dead white blood cells)—called hypopyon—at the bottom of the anterior chamber, a telltale sign of inflammation.

My heart sank.

Whenever we saw hypopyon, it was always an emergency.

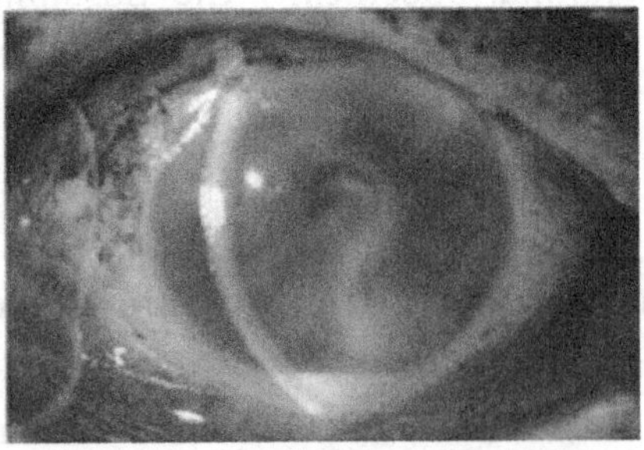

Hypopyon: the yellow layer of pus at the bottom of the anterior chamber

Endophthalmitis is inflammation of the interior cavity of the eye, usually caused by infection. It is a possible complication of all intraocular surgeries, particularly cataract surgery, and can result in loss of vision or loss of the eye itself. Infection can be caused by bacteria or fungi, and is classified as exogenous or endogenous. Other non-infectious causes include toxins, allergic reactions and retained intraocular foreign bodies.

We needed to find out what was causing the inflammation as quickly as possible. It could be sterile, meaning it was a reaction to the surgery or some drugs used. If that were the case, then corticosteroids would be needed to decrease or stop the inflammation.

The most common cause of endophthalmitis is bacterial. Many different kinds of bacteria can cause such inflammation. Some don't cause severe damage; but some, like pseudomonas, could destroy the eye in a matter of a day or two.

Another cause of inflammation could be fungus. If so, then we had to treat it with anti-fungal drugs.

Seeing the concern on my face, Mrs. Hamilton asked, "Something wrong, Dr. Hung?"

"There's quite a bit of inflammation in the eye," I responded. "We have to find out what's causing it. I'm concerned that it could be caused by bacteria or fungus. To find out, I need to do some tests. I need to take a little fluid from your eye and send it to the lab for analysis. It won't hurt," I reassured her.

I instilled a few drops of Lidocaine on her eye. With a tiny needle, I aspirated a small amount of the fluid from the vitreous cavity and did the usual procedure, smearing the sample on a glass slide and placing the sample in a culture medium.

"While we're waiting for the results, I'd like to give you a small amount of antibiotics in the eye," I said. "If the inflammation turns out to be caused by bacteria, you'd be covered. If not, no harm done. But time is of the essence," I explained to Mrs. Hamilton and her daughter.

I again instilled a few more drop of the Lidocaine on her eye, and with a quick stab, I injected a small amount of a broad-spectrum antibiotic (vancomycin) into her vitreous cavity.

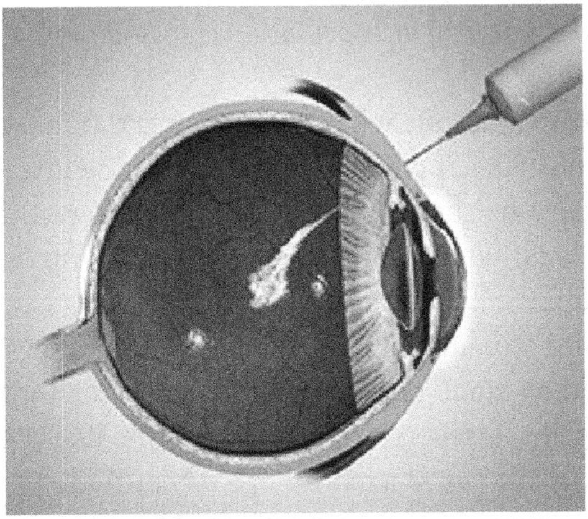

Injecting antibiotics inside the eye

"Because it could be fast-growing bacteria, we need to admit you to the hospital to give you IV antibiotics around the clock, and to monitor you closely. I am sorry for the inconvenience," I said.

"Things happen," said Mrs. Hamilton, as if she was trying to console me.

The following day, a Saturday, the lab results came back. The inflammation was caused by a bacterium called staphylococcus epidermidis, i.e., from the skin.

The culture and sensitivity tests of the bacteria showed that it was sensitive to vancomycin. It just happened that the small amount of antibiotic I'd injected into Mrs. Hamilton's eye was vancomycin and the IV antibiotic she'd been getting was vancomycin as well.

I examined Mrs. Hamilton carefully, and was relieved to see that the inflammation in her eye was definitely not any worse, and perhaps even a little bit better. She was more comfortable, but her vision was still blurry, about 20/100.

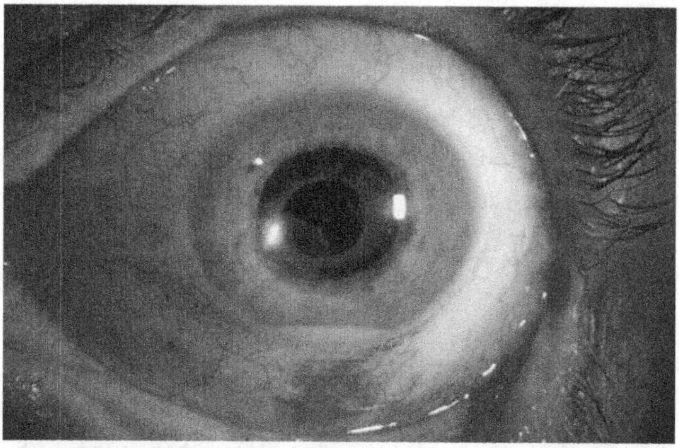

The inflammation in her eye was a little bit better

"I'm very sorry that you have to be in the hospital," I said apologetically. "I don't understand how you came down with this infection. Last night, I went over the video of your surgery and everything went so well. I can't think of anything that would have caused this. We know that there are bacteria everywhere, and this one seems to be from a person's skin. The lab tests show that we're using the right antibiotic."

"Dr. Hung, things happen," Mrs. Hamilton said again. "I have confidence in you and I'm sure that the infection will go away and my eye will be alright." Again, I got the feeling that she was trying to reassure me instead of the other way around. She knew how upset I was.

"I'll see you tomorrow," I continued, "but I'm leaving on Monday for London for an eye meeting that was planned over a year ago. Dr. Mendoza, my associate, will take care of you while I'm gone. I will talk to him daily," I added.

After examining her, I said, "The infection is definitely getting better." Her visual acuity had improved to 20/80. "The pus inside your eye, which we call hypopyon, is almost all gone."

"Yes, I'm definitely feeling better," Mrs. Hamilton said with a smile. "The ache is gone, and I can see better today."

Monday morning I flew to London. The following day, I called Mrs. Hamilton at the hospital. She was surprised to hear from me. I told her that Dr. Mendoza had reported to me that she continued to improve.

I called her again the next day.

"Dr. Hung, please don't worry," she exclaimed. "I'll be alright. Enjoy your meeting."

When I talked to Dr. Mendoza again, he said Mrs. Hamilton felt very bad that I was so worried about her.

I returned a week later. Mrs. Hamilton was out of the hospital, her infection had disappeared and her vision was 20/25.

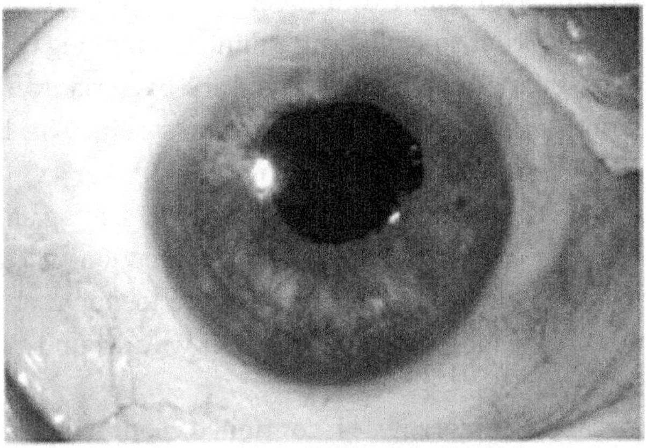

The infection had cleared
Vision was 20/25.

On a Tuesday morning, Mrs. Hamilton came into the office for follow-up.

With a big smile on her face, she gave me a hug and said, "I really felt bad that you were so worried about me."

"Thank you," I said. "I'm glad everything turned out alright."

From my years of taking care of patients, I've learnt that most patients are reasonable, kind and understanding. If they feel that their doctor is doing his or her best, that they're being told the truth, and that the doctor is truly concerned about them, they will forgive the doctor even if a mistake is made.

Looking back at Mrs. Hamilton's case almost thirty years later, I think it's ironic that when things weren't going well, she was feeling bad that her doctor was so worried about her instead of being upset about the complication itself.

Chapter 29
Xinjiang

RECENTLY THE UYGHUR PEOPLE have been in the news again. It was reported that since 2017 the Chinese government has locked up over one million Uyghurs in re-educational camps. I was distressed to learn that these people were still being mistreated in China. The people and culture have always fascinated me.

In 1996, I was again headed for Guilin in southwest China to help the People's Number Two Hospital set up a laser machine for the treatment of different retinal conditions. On the way, I stopped in Beijing for a couple of days to make the plane connection.

At the Great Wall Sheraton Hotel in Beijing, I was browsing the lobby bookstore and came across an old book entitled *An English Lady in Chinese Turkestan*. It was about an English woman named Catherine Borland, who at age 21 married George Macartney, Britain's representative at Kashgar from 1890 to 1918. The author, Lady Macartney, wrote about her life in Kashgar, which at the time was one of the most remote and desolate places on earth.

The description of her journey from England to Kashgar was fascinating. It took many months and began with a train from London across Europe, through Russia, over the Caspian Sea, and along the trans-Caspian railway to Andijan in present-day Uzbekistan. From Andijan to Osh—in present-day Kyrgyzstan—the journey continued in a slow, uncomfortable post cart; and from Osh to Kashgar, the party climbed over the Tian-Shan Mountains on horseback. The book impressed upon me how difficult and dangerous traveling was in those days, and prompted me to go ahead with my lifelong wish to visit Xinjiang and make plans to see the house where Lady Macartney had lived in Kashgar.

After reading her book, I decided to learn more about the Uyghur people, who made up the majority of the population in the Xinjiang area.

The history of the Uyghur people is complicated. From various sources, it is generally accepted that the original Uyghurs were part of a Turkic confederation that lived in the valleys south of Lake Baikal. In 840, following a civil war and famine, the Kyrgyz—another Turkic people—defeated them. These Uyghurs moved south and eventually settled in the Turpan area in Xinjiang. They abandoned nomadism and began farming.

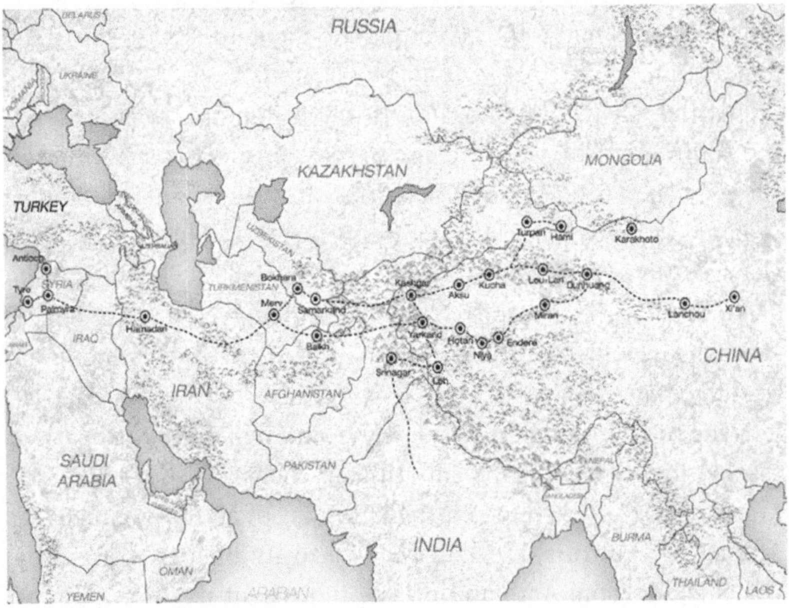

The Silk Road, home of most of the Turkic people

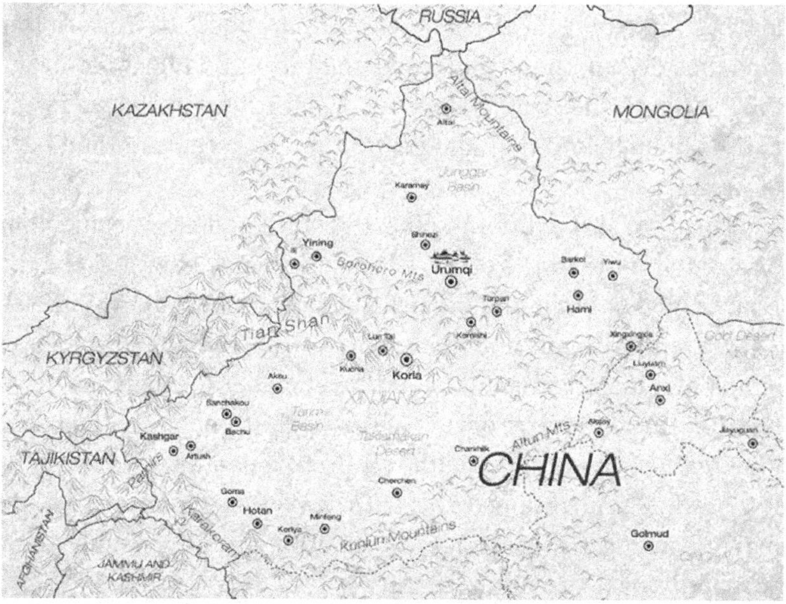

Xinjiang, China, home of the Uyghurs

So who is a Uyghur? It's generally agreed that a Uyghur is a Turkic person who speaks the Uyghur language—one of the 30 Turkic languages—and who is not a Kazakh, Uzbek, Kyrgyz, Tajik or Tartar, and certainly not a Han. A Uyghur's identity is determined by one's family history.

With the tremendous advancements in genetics, various studies have shown that the Uyghurs are a Eurasian population with Eastern and Western Eurasian genetic traits. They are one of the many populations of Central Eurasia that can be considered genetically related to both East Asian and European populations. In one study, using samples from Hotan in the south (also known as Hetian or Khotan), Uyghurs were found to have 60% European genes.

China has had dealings in Xinjiang for thousands of years. In 1949, when the communists took over China, the Uyghur language was switched to the Latin alphabet. When Deng

Xiaoping adopted a more open policy in the 1970s, the Uyghur leaders in Xinjiang decided to switch back to the Arabic alphabet. (When the Uyghurs switched from Buddhism to Islam, they adopted the Arabic alphabet. Then it was switched to the Latin alphabet, and then to Cyrillic, then to Latin, and then back to Arabic.)

This explains why, in some Uyghur families, one member often can't write to the other, because one may have learned the Latin alphabet while the other had learned the Arabic alphabet. There's a movement underway now to switch back to the Latin alphabet. I feel that using the Arabic alphabet for their language is a hindrance to the progress of the Uyghur people, and most of my Uyghur friends agree with me. From a personal perspective, I wish they had retained the Latin alphabet because it would make learning the language easier. The Arabic alphabet adds another barrier to communication.

So much of the history of this region was confusing to me, and yet fascinating at the same time. The picture was becoming clearer about the origin of the Uyghur people and the other minorities living in Xinjiang. I hoped that by being better informed, I could understand these people better and make my experience in Xinjiang more meaningful.

In 2000, I made my first trip to Xinjiang and gave a workshop on using the indirect ophthalmoscope, which was new to China at that point, to all the ophthalmologists in the province at the government-run Urumqi City Eye Hospital. At this workshop, I met a charismatic Uyghur woman named Dr. Adiya.

Realizing the needs of her people, and with her own financial resources, she had opened her own eye clinic called the Adiya Eye Hospital, mainly to serve the Uyghur people. Many of them were poor and couldn't afford to pay for the services.

I was invited to visit the clinic, which was in south Urumqi. While I was there, Dr. Adiya asked me to assess a man in his fifties who had come from the distant south, even further than Hotan, whose right eye had been blinded by a local shaman. His left eye now also had a dense cataract and he was hoping Dr. Adiya could help him.

This poor man had a procedure done by the shaman called "couching," which involved using the finger or an instrument to apply pressure on the eyeball, causing the cataractous lens to be pushed away from its support and fall to the back of the eye into the vitreous. This procedure worked some of the time, but often the lens in the vitreous caused severe inflammation and eventually led to blindness.

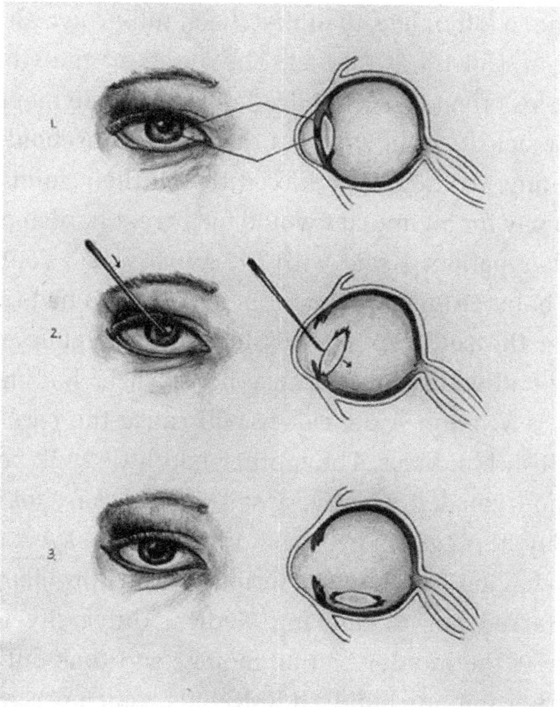

Couching is an ancient method of cataract treatment whereby the cataractous lens is dislocated from the visual axis into the vitreous cavity. It is the first documented form of cataract treatment. It was thought to have been first invented in India 800 years BC during the Sushruta period.

I was so surprised that this ancient procedure was still being done in Xinjiang. There was nothing Dr. Adiya could do for the blind eye, but she could remove the cataract from the other eye. I offered to pay for the patient's implant, and promised that when I returned, I would bring two hundred IOLs from the company I had dealt with in Virginia in the US.

Cataracts are more common in the desert because the people are exposed to long hours of strong sunlight.

The level of poverty in rural Xinjiang was beyond my imagination. Often, all a family had was a hut, a small plot of land for growing vegetables and fruits and a herd of perhaps some twenty sheep, often less than that. Each full-grown sheep would bring about $50 US at market. The assets of the whole family would be less than a few hundred dollars. If one member of the family got sick, it could wipe out the entire household savings, if they had any, or they were forced to sell their animals. Simply having to pay for an implant would be a great hardship.

Another patient I saw with Dr. Adiya was a young mother with her baby girl of three months old. She too had traveled for days from the south to see this legendary Uyghur eye doctor. The baby had gone blind because her corneas had melted. In a newborn, a Vitamin A deficiency will cause the cornea to melt and result in blindness. The mother had little milk because she was malnourished. It was a very sad sight because for only a few cents a day, this baby's eyes could have been saved. The infant was also having other more serious health problems and Dr. Adiya referred her to Xinjiang Medical University for further care. I knew the mother had no money, so I took out my wallet and gave her ten one hundred RMB bills, which was a little over $100 US. I wish I had more money with me that day.

I reminded myself that this was China's problem and it was not my place to solve the country's difficulties. It was a matter of the government setting its priorities. Up to that point, I had been quite good about not being distracted by other issues, and simply focused on what I could do. But seeing a newborn blind because the family couldn't afford a few cents a day for Vitamin A had an effect on me that lasted for weeks, the image of the blind baby etched in my mind. I thought about how wonderful it would be if I could take care of the mother and baby, and later help the baby with her education, making sure she had decent opportunities in life. I reminded myself that there were millions of such people, and there was no way I could help every one of them. So many of them were in such dire situations due to circumstances beyond their control.

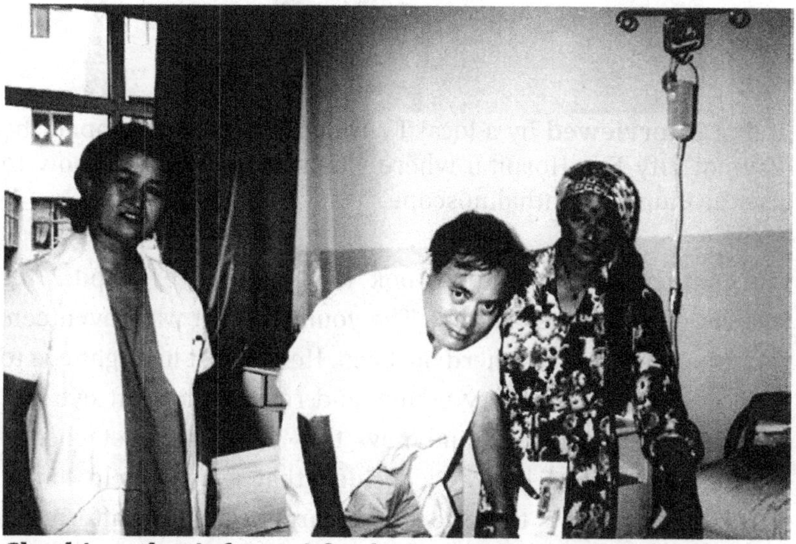

Checking the infant girl whose corneas melted because of Vitamin A deficiency. Dr. Adiya is on the left. On the right is the baby's mother who had traveled for days from Hotan, a distant oasis town in the south of the province. The baby was referred to the university hospital as she had numerous medical problems in addition to her eyes.

I usually didn't let the patients get to me, but sometimes they just did. In a childish way, I imagined how good it would feel if I could solve everyone's problems. As a child I envied Superman and wished I had his super powers that enabled him to do things others couldn't. I still had such fantasies.

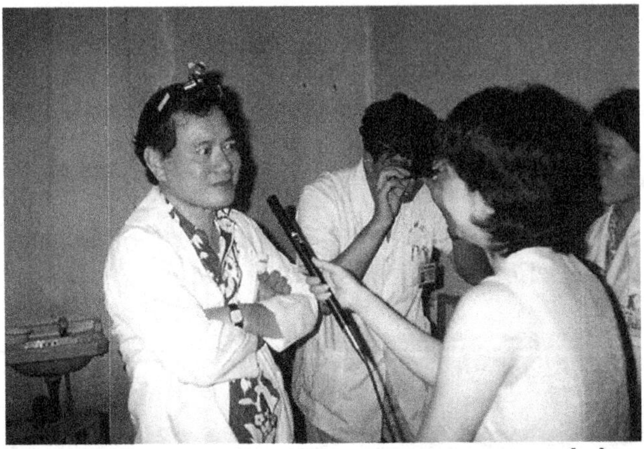

Being interviewed by a local TV reporter at a workshop at the Urumqi City Eye Hospital where I taught local doctors how to use the indirect ophthalmoscope.

On another day, Dr. Adiya took me to her eye hospital for evaluation of another patient. The young patient was seventeen, a farmer who tended a herd of sheep. He had lost his right eye to a rock when he was very young, and recently his left eye had been struck by a stick and now the retina had detached. I carefully examined him and decided that I could help him. I made arrangements to perform the surgery the next afternoon, as I already had a surgery scheduled at the Urumqi Eye Hospital in the north of the city for the morning.

I felt very fortunate to have selected ophthalmology and especially retina surgery, because it was something few people could do, and it often saved people's eyesight. I was proud to offer my services overseas, because most of the time I could help patients who might not have access to such a specialist otherwise. The eye, unlike some other parts of the body, could be examined and treated whether the patient was a man or woman, regardless of country, culture or religion; there was nothing taboo about the eye.

The morning surgery at the Urumqi Eye Hospital was for a thirty-year-old woman from Kashgar in the southwest of the province. It took her and her husband three days on the bus to get there. The husband hung around the hospital during the day and slept wherever he could during the night because they had no money for a hotel. The patient's detached retina was in the upper half of her right eye, and it only took me a little over an hour to complete the surgery, in spite of working in an unfamiliar place. It helped that I had brought my own surgical instruments.

The surgery went very well. The hole in the retina that had caused the detachment was easily treated and closed. The retina hadn't been detached for very long—at the most one week—which also made it easier to re-attach.

At the end of the surgery, the retina was fully attached.

Dr. Adiya had a full clinic of patients that morning at her own hospital and was unable to come observe me in surgery at the city-run hospital. She had her brother, a custodian at the clinic, come fetch me in her car. We had a quick lunch in the dining room and then went to work. Her eye hospital was much smaller than the Urumqi Eye Hospital, but she did three times the number of surgeries each week.

The young man's detached retina was very thin, almost transparent, indicating that it had been detached for some time. There were several holes in the retina, which made the repair more difficult. It was a much more challenging operation than the one I'd done that morning, but it was finished without complication. Dr. Adiya assisted me.

The next morning I checked on both patients and was pleased that the surgeries had been successful. The woman's vision was 20/25. The young man's vision was 20/200, but because the retina had been detached for a while, it would take longer for the vision to improve. In some cases, it might not improve because the damage done by having the retina separated from the underlying layers was permanent. Sometimes the body couldn't repair the damaged retinal cells; but I was hopeful that with time the young farmer's vision would improve.

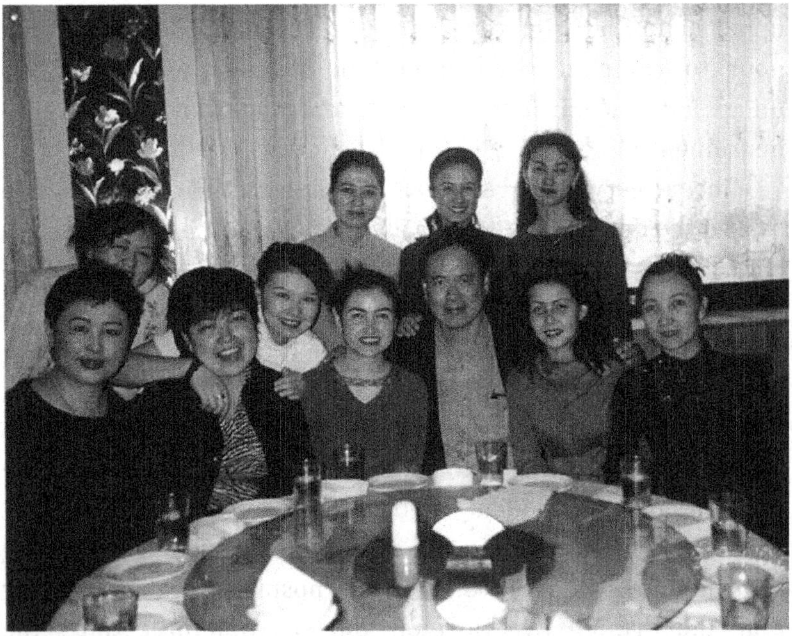

Employees of the Adiya Eye Hospital: nurses, assistants, cleaners, etc. Almost all of them are Uyghurs with the exception of the woman whose face is partially hidden in the second row. She is Han Chinese.

Behind me, with her hand on my shoulder, is the excellent surgical technician Elmira. Standing to her left is Alina, who is in charge of the Optical Shop. To her right is Patigul, an assistant in the clinic who is also a professional folk dancer.

I'm very glad that I made the effort to help the people in Xinjiang. Instead of working day after day in my office—days that I might hardly remember—now I can remember all the things I did in Xinjiang. I can also recall almost every man, woman and child I met there.

My life has been enriched greatly because of those trips.

Chapter 30
Is Life Happenstance?

AIRPLANE CRASHES ARE USUALLY VERY RARE, but in 1987, there were three within a two-week period. The newspaper headlines read:

- November 28, 1987: South African Airways Flight 295 crashes into the Indian Ocean, killing all 159 people on board.
- November 29, 1987: Korean Air Flight 858 explodes over the Thai–Burmese border, killing 115.
- December 7, 1987: Pacific Southwest Airlines Flight 1771 crashes near Paso Robles, California, killing all 43 on board, after a disgruntled ex-employee shoots his ex-boss traveling on the flight, then shoots both pilots and himself.

It seems that things do come in threes. Within a matter of ten days in the last part of 1987, the three plane crashes claimed over 300 lives.

In Chinese culture, people believe in karma. They believe that when something bad happens to someone, it's because that person—or his or her ancestors—have done something bad, hence the karmic retribution.

But how does one explain these 300 deaths? How could it be possible that all of them or their ancestors had done something bad?

People's fate, good luck and bad luck have always intrigued me. Most cultures have their own way of trying to make sense of bad fortune, untimely deaths and other tragedies. Whenever I treated someone with a bad problem, I often wondered why it had to happen to this poor patient.

It was about this time that I treated three people with horrific eye injuries to the eye. One was lucky, and the other two were not.

It was the last week of December. The weather had gotten cold in Fresno. I could see people's chimney smoke coming from their fireplaces. Even though burning wood in the San Joaquin Valley caused horrible pollution because the particulates got trapped in the valley by the fog, people still continued burning wood fires.

After dinner one evening, I got a call from the ER doc at the hospital saying that a woman had come in with something in her eye. Apparently she was sitting by the fire at home when she heard an explosion in the fireplace, followed by a sharp pain in her eye and cloudy vision.

"You mean, she got a piece of metal inside her eye?" I asked.

"I think so but I can't see anything," the ER doc replied.

"I'll come in," I said.

When I arrived at the ER, an attractive woman in her early thirties was sitting there with a man of about the same age, and a young boy of about five. The woman had a shield over her left eye.

I introduced myself and learned that the patient's name was Wanda Whitman. She seemed a little uncomfortable and reported that she had a deep ache in her eye.

"What happened?" I asked.

"We were sitting by the fireplace watching TV," Wanda explained. "All of a sudden, I heard a bang from the fireplace, then I felt something hot hit my left eye, then I saw dark spots."

"What do you think hit you?" I asked.

"I'm not sure," she replied, shaking her head. "We don't have any guns or bullets at home. But I don't know what was in the firewood. It could have been something in the wood that exploded."

Examination of Wanda's left eye showed no obvious leak and the pressure of the eyeball seemed normal. There was hemorrhage inside the eye, but I couldn't see any metallic object.

"I see blood at the 3 o'clock position inside your eye," I told Wanda. "The blood could be obscuring the metal. We need to do some X-rays."

Once the films were available, I could see a small piece of metal at the 3 o'clock position in the sclera. I couldn't tell how deep it was or if it had hit the retina.

I explained to Wanda and her husband that she needed surgery to get the piece of metal out. As I couldn't tell how deep the metal was, I didn't know how extensive the surgery would be.

Since Wanda's eye didn't seem to be leaking any fluid, I decided that surgery could wait till the next day. She was admitted to the hospital and given IV antibiotics to prevent infection.

I did the surgery the next morning. Wanda was very fortunate that the piece of metal hit her eye in that particular area, and had narrowly missed the lens and retina. The metal landed in the *pars plana*, an area in the eye that didn't have many blood vessels and consisted mostly of connective tissue.

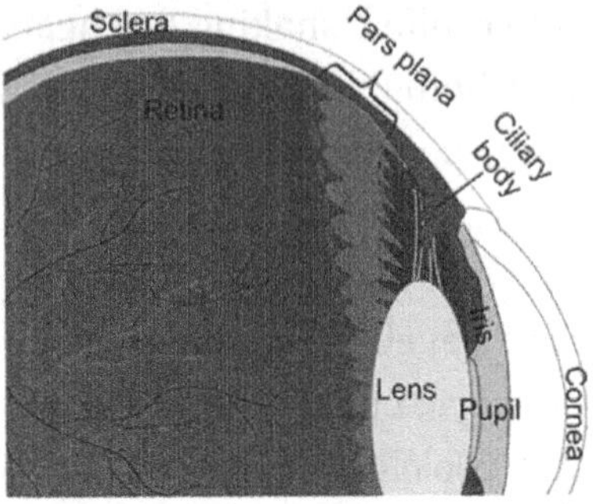

Pars plana is an area inside the eye that has few blood vessels and is actually where we make incisions when we do a vitrectomy and where we insert different instruments into the eye.

With a strong magnet, the tiny fragment of metal was removed. After I removed the metal, there was a small leakage of fluid. I closed the wound with two sutures, and the leak stopped.

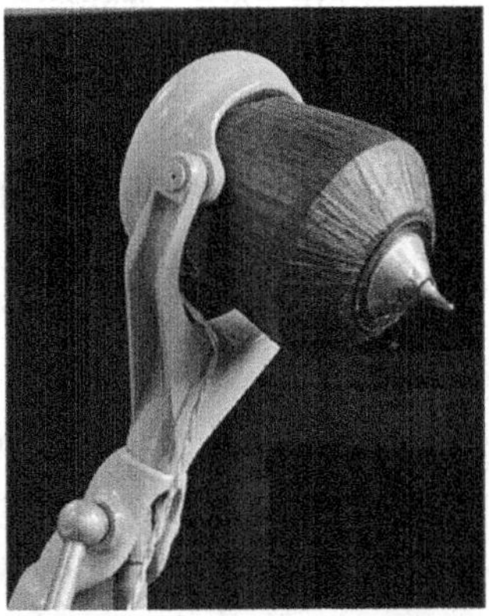

A powerful magnet for use in eye surgery, specifically designed to remove metallic foreign bodies in or on the eye. This one was commonly used in 1987, but the instrument has been improved over the years. The size of the magnet has decreased, while its power has increased.

I examined Wanda's eye again, but I couldn't tell if she had any retina tearing from the entry wound because of the blood obscuring the area. To be safe, I treated the sclera around the area where the piece of metal had hit with cryo therapy to make sure that any possible retina tear was treated.

Wanda healed well. The hemorrhage in her left eye soon disappeared and her vision returned to 20/20. The eye had healed so well that it was as if she'd never had any surgery. This was a very happy ending.

Later, I learned that Wanda was the San Joaquin Valley's ice skating queen.

"Thank you so much Dr. Hung," she said at her follow up exam. "I'm glad you saved my eye—it would be difficult for me to skate with one eye," she joked.

She was truly fortunate that the metal didn't enter her eye. If it had, trying to get it out would have been much more difficult and would have involved a major surgery such as vitrectomy. If the metal had gone 1 mm deeper or more posteriorly, or anteriorly, the injury would have been more severe and the prognosis not as good.

Wanda was very lucky in an unlucky situation.

***

A few days later, on a Friday afternoon, I received a call from Dr. Schuman at his Workmen's Comp Clinic to say that he was referring a patient to me with an eye injury caused by baling wire.

Otis Brown was a sixty-year-old farm worker. He had been trying to cut the wire on a bale of hay to feed the animals when the wire snapped and recoiled, hitting him in the right eye. He felt a sharp pain, followed by a gush of fluid and blood from that eye.

Examination of his right eye showed that it was covered by a large blood clot. I could barely see the cornea. I touched the eye gently with a sterile cotton tip applicator and noted that it was soft, indicating a wound that was leaking.

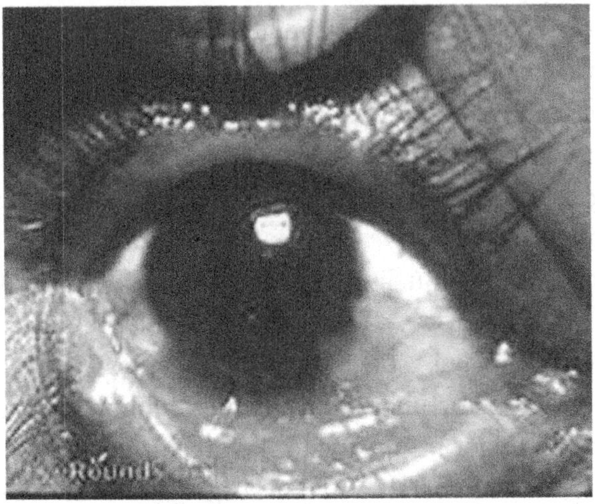

Baling wire eye injury

An injury like Otis' was an emergency. I sent him to the hospital to start IV antibiotics and got him ready for surgery as soon as possible. As Otis hadn't eaten lunch, we were able to do the surgery that day, as soon as I finished seeing the patients in my clinic.

In the operating room, Otis was put to sleep and I was able to carefully examine the severely injured eye. I carefully removed the large blood clot and irrigated the area with copious amounts of saline. Soon, the cornea was visible. It had a large wound. The baling wire had cut Otis' cornea into two halves. The wound extended posteriorly, involving the sclera. It was a large injury involving multiple important structures in the eye.

I couldn't find the lens in his eye, and I concluded that it must have been extruded through the large corneal wound. The iris was prolapsed through the wound, and there were other grayish tissues also protruding from it. It was a horrendous injury.

At that point, my goal was to save the eye. Whether we could save his sight was another matter. Some ophthalmologists would actually remove the eye at this point because of the danger of Sympathetic Ophthalmia.

Sympathetic Ophthalmia (SO) is a rare, bilateral, severe inflammation of the eye caused by injury to one eye. It's believed to be an autoimmune inflammatory response to ocular antigens. Immunosuppressive therapy with corticosteroid is the main treatment.

From my experience, most patients would be devastated waking up from anesthesia to be told their eye had been removed. Usually, no matter how bad the injury was, I always tried to save the eye and then discuss the possibility of removing it with the patient later. People needed time to make such a difficult decision.

Otis was a stoic man and never complained about his injury.

"Doc, just do what you have to do," he would tell me.

After three surgeries involving reconstruction of his eye, to my surprise, Otis' vision improved to 20/200, which was legally blind but still a lot better than losing that eye. With 20/200 vision, a person would be able to get around and take care of himself or herself.

A year later, Otis was comfortable and free from any discomfort in his eye. The left eye showed an obvious grayish-white scar on the cornea, which Otis claimed didn't bother him.

I advised him to always wear protective glasses to make sure that his good eye was protected.

Why did such an injury have to happen? If Otis had worn safety glasses, that piece of wire never would have touched his eye. If he had followed safety guidelines when cutting the wire, such as keeping a safe distance, that eye wouldn't have been hit. In that split second, Otis essentially lost the use of his eye; and even though he still retained the eye, he was basically depending only on his good eye. It was just bad luck that this horrible injury happened to Otis.

***

A few days after I met Otis, on New Year's Eve, shortly after midnight, I got a call from the ER doctor at the hospital reporting that they had a man there who had suffered severe injuries to his right eye from a firecracker.

When I arrived at the ER, I found a man in his mid-thirties in obvious pain. His right eye was covered by a large blood clot. I couldn't even see the eye. I noted some grayish tissue extruding from the eye mixed with the blood clot. I touched the eye gently with a sterile cotton tip applicator and it was soft.

Ken Worth was a firefighter from Walnut Creek in the San Francisco Bay Area who had come to Fresno to celebrate New Year's Eve with his cousin. They were at a party and someone threw a large firecracker, which exploded in front of Ken's face.

This firecracker turned out to be a cherry bomb, commonly referred to as M-80s and quarter sticks. These were illegal firecrackers that contained a large amount of explosives and were extremely dangerous.

There was no way to assess the damage with Ken awake. We quickly assembled a surgical team and got him into the OR.

After the large blood clot was removed, it revealed an eye that looked like a squashed grape. The wound was jagged. The lens was missing. Trapped in the large wound was part of the iris and what looked like retina tissue.

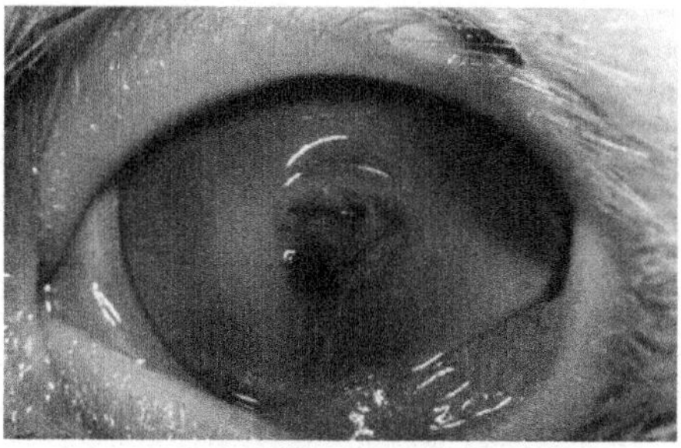

Firecracker eye injury

This was a catastrophic injury. It was obvious that there was little chance of saving the eye, but still I chose not to remove it, to allow Ken more time to adjust to the loss of such an important part of his body.

Loss of the eye, I was told, was different from the loss of other body parts, because we see ourselves with our eyes, and we're constantly reminded of the loss.

I carefully reconstructed Ken's eye, suturing the large wound as well as I could, and trying to salvage as much tissue as possible. In the end, the eye was watertight and showed no leakage anywhere.

The following day, I explained to Ken and his family what I had done and that, because of the very severe injury, it was unlikely that any sight could be saved.

As he lived in the San Francisco area, I recommended that he be followed up near his home, saying that I'd be happy to refer him to the University of California San Francisco Medical Center.

A few months later, I received a letter from Ken's lawyer requesting a deposition from me about the extent of his injuries. Ken was suing the owner of the home where the party was held. I never found out if they caught whoever threw the cherry bomb.

Such is the fate of us humans. Ken was in the wrong place at the wrong time, and in the matter of a split second, he lost his eye.

I later learned that Ken had that eye removed and was fitted with a porcelain eye. He could no longer work as a firefighter.

Ken would not have lost the eye:

- If he had celebrated the New Year at home!
- If he had arrived at the party a second sooner or later!
- If he had not stood in that very spot!
- If he had worn glasses, the injury might not have been as severe!

That's just how life is. You never know what's waiting for you around the corner.

Chapter 31
House Calls

"A physician's experience goes far beyond the clinical, because a person is never merely a disease, a disorder of biology. Each interaction between a doctor and a patient is a story."

I'VE ALWAYS REMEMBERED THIS SAYING by William Carlos Williams, one of my favorite writers. He wrote much about his house calls, which I enjoyed reading tremendously. Each time I saw an older patient, I often wondered what sort of life he or she had lived, and what sort of life he or she was living now.

One of my patients was an elderly Armenian man who had been under my care for over a year. He had a difficult case of glaucoma that hadn't responded to any sorts of drops. The next step would be to do a delicate procedure called trabeculectomy. These were the days before laser treatment was used for glaucoma.

Trabeculectomy is a type of glaucoma surgery that creates a new pathway for fluid inside the eye to be drained. It's designed to prevent worsening of vision loss by lowering eye pressure.

When performing trabeculectomy, an eye surgeon creates a flap in the sclera—the white part of the eye. The drainage pathway is created under this flap, and the flap is then placed loosely back down against the sclera to protect the new pathway. Finally, the entire surgery site is covered up using the outermost covering of the eye (the conjunctiva).

This process results in a small blister of fluid, called a bleb, on top of the eye's surface but underneath the eyelid. The fluid inside the blister gets absorbed into blood vessels. The bleb is hidden by the upper eyelid and generally not noticeable by other people.

Trabeculectomy doesn't restore vision that's already been lost. The purpose of the procedure is just to prevent further loss of vision due to glaucoma.

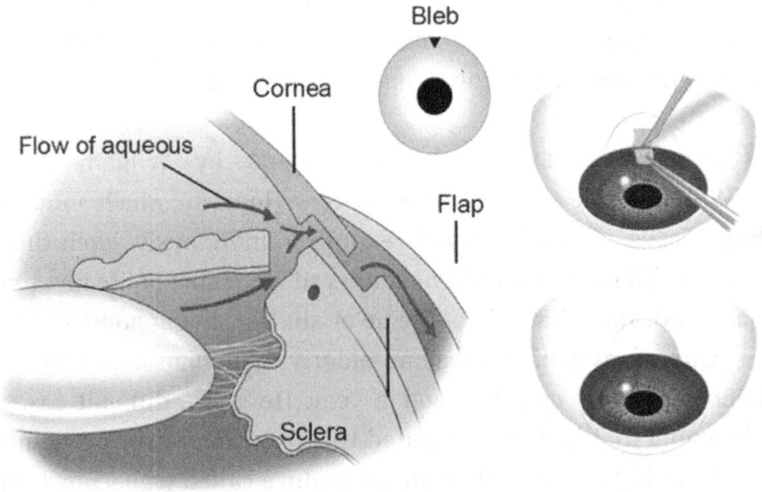

Trabeculectomy

Mr. Hajibian was a slight man, with deep wrinkles all over his small, narrow face. The top of his head was completely bald, and the remaining hair on the sides and back of his head was white. He had intense dark brown eyes, covered partially by loose upper eyelids. He always had a worried look on his face.

He was a man of few words, but I could tell that he liked and trusted me. He always came to the office alone, and from what I learned, he always took the bus. In the Fresno summer heat of over 100°F, it must have been very uncomfortable.

On Mr. Hajibian's surgery day, everything went as planned. Trabeculectomy is one of the most unpredictable and challenging eye surgeries, as we hope the small opening will drain just the right amount to give the eye a pressure that won't damage the optic nerve further. If the opening drains too much, the pressure in the eye is too low, and the cornea could touch the iris or, worse, the lens, which would cause the formation of a cataract. Adhesions could also form between the lens and iris if the pressure in the eye is too low. On the other hand, if the opening doesn't drain enough, the pressure remains elevated and the surgery was a failure.

I was pleased that Mr. Hajibian's surgery went well, and I asked one of my office assistants to take him home once we were finished. As he had no relatives, getting to and from the office was a hardship, especially following eye surgery, and Mr. Hajibian couldn't afford taxi fare. This was before the now ubiquitous transportation for seniors.

Before he left, I told him that I'd like to visit him at his home the following day after work.

The next day, a Friday, I was finished with all my patients by 5 pm and I headed for Mr. Hajibian's home in south Fresno. It was a nondescript one-bedroom apartment with spartan furnishings.

Mr. Hajibian was very pleased to see me and had a big smile on his face as he showed me into his apartment.

"Thanks for coming, Doc. I really appreciate it," he said.

"I'm happy to do it. How are you feeling?" I asked.

"There's a little ache, but otherwise I think I feel all right," he answered.

Walking slowly with his right eye patched, he brought me a cup and began to pour dark brown tea into it.

I took the cup and thanked him, and then when he was settled with his own tea, I asked, "How long have you lived in Fresno?"

"Doc, it's a long story," Mr. Hajibian sighed.

"Before you begin your story, do you mind if I check your eye first?"

"Of course," he replied, setting down his cup.

While he sat on his couch, I removed the eye shield and then the eye patch underneath it. I put on my head-mounted microscope with a light source, and looked into his right eye. I then instilled a few drops of Lidocaine in his eye and gently touched the eyeball with a sterile cotton tip applicator. The pressure felt a little soft, but the cornea was away from the iris, which was what we wanted.

"So far so good," I reported. "The pressure is below 10, which is great at this stage. As the eye heals, the pressure should slowly get higher. We hope it stays below 15. That would be ideal."

I applied an ointment to the eye and placed a new eye patch, then covered it with the same eye shield.

I was very relieved that things looked good.

"So," I said, putting my microscope and supplies back into my bag, "we were talking about how you ended up in Fresno."

"It's a long story," Mr. Hajibian repeated.

I smiled and said, "I'm always interested to hear my patient's life story."

"Well," he began, "you probably don't know about the Armenian genocide by the Turks."

"I do," I replied. "I've had a number of my Armenian patients tell me about how they escaped and ended up in Fresno."

The Armenian genocide refers to the physical annihilation of Armenian Christian people living in the Ottoman Empire from the spring of 1915 through the autumn of 1916. Over one million Armenians perished or were murdered during the death marches to the Syrian Desert. Armenian women and children were forced to convert to Islam.

Mr. Hajibian nodded and continued. "My parents were dead. My brother and I walked for days before arriving in Damascus in present-day Syria. Somehow we survived. My brother Hagop was twenty and I was fifteen. Hagop was eventually able to get in touch with some relatives in New York City and they sponsored us to immigrate to America.

"We arrived in New York City in 1920, when I was twenty years old. The people who sponsored us had a carpet shop in Mid-Manhattan, and both my brother and I helped in the shop and learned the trade.

"When I found out that one of my uncles lived in Fresno and owned a large farm and a packinghouse, I thought I would like to live in an environment that reminded me of the old country. My relatives wrote that Fresno was much like Armenia.

"I moved here and worked in the packinghouse for many years. Unfortunately I wasn't able to save much money and I never married. When I retired ten years ago, all I had was social security, which was only a few hundred dollars a month. So, this is all I can afford," he said, gesturing to the apartment.

"Perhaps I should have stayed in New York," he added thoughtfully. "Perhaps I should have gotten married. Perhaps I should have learnt a trade. Perhaps I should have gotten more education." He sighed and paused to refill our tea cups.

"The worst thing is to be short on money all the time," he continued. "I'm on a wait list for the California Armenian Home—my life would be safer there. I wouldn't have to cook and they provide transportation to the doctor's office."

I mostly listened, and occasionally asked a question. I was sad to see this 80-year-old man so full of regrets, wondering if he should have done this or that. I found his story fascinating, and I wondered how many other people his age had as many regrets as him.

It was evident that Mr. Hajibian was very pleased with my house call and to have someone to talk to.

I stayed until we'd finished the pot of tea.

"So far so good," I said again as I was leaving. "I'd like to come check on you again tomorrow. Do you need anything from the store?" I asked.

"Doc, if it's not too much trouble, could you please get some bananas, milk, bacon, eggs and a loaf of whole wheat bread," he replied.

"No problem," I reassured him. "I'm more than happy to do it."

The following day, a Saturday, at noon, I stopped by the grocery store and got what Mr. Hajibian needed. He was very happy to see me and again had a big smile on his face. It was the first time I'd seen him smile so widely. He always seemed so serious, his eyebrows always narrowed, when I saw him in my office.

I again examined his eye. The pressure had gone up slightly which was what we wanted. There was no sign of infection or any other complications. We were both very pleased with how the eye was healing.

Again, he made a pot of tea and we talked.

"Mr. Hajibian, do you know how your parents died?" I asked.

"I was really young so I don't know the details," he answered. "But my brother Hagop told me that they died of starvation, along with tens of thousands of other Armenians after they were driven from their homes and marched for weeks in the desert, without food, trying to escape to wherever they could—Iran, Iraq, Lebanon, Syria, and some far-away places like Argentina.

"I think most of the Armenians in Fresno have done well, except for a few people like me," he sighed.

"Don't be too hard on yourself," I said, trying to sound optimistic. "You're 80 and you have your health. I guess we all want more money to live more comfortably.

"Mr. Hajibian, I'm really glad that I visited you. I've learnt so much," I said. I was truly fascinated hearing about his life.

I bid him goodbye and told him that I'd like to see him again the following day. If he continued to do well, I wouldn't have to see him for another week.

In the end, Mr. Hajibian's eye healed just right, and the pressure was twelve, which was excellent. With that kind of pressure, his eye wouldn't lose anymore visual field.

A few months later, he told me that his application to the Armenian Home was approved, and he'd been living there for the past month. He was pleased with the living conditions, and happy that he could speak his language again, eat the kind of food he liked and have many people to talk to.

***

Slim Allred was quite the opposite of Mr. Hajibian. Perhaps when he was young he'd been a skinny boy, but at age 70, he was over six feet tall and weighed over 200 pounds. There was nothing slim about Mr. Allred.

Slim had worked as a long haul truck driver since he was in his mid-twenties. Now with poorly controlled hypertension, and after a minor stroke, he'd moved into an assisted care facility named *Twilight Haven*. I thought it was such a poor name for a place that housed people who were literally living out their twilight years. It seemed to me like one of the most inappropriate names for a nursing home.

Slim was a big man, with a big, round, bald head. He spoke with an accent that I was now familiar with, the Okie accent. He wasn't a very friendly man, and he didn't talk much.

He was referred to me because of bleeding in his right eye as well as cataracts in both eyes. He was no longer able to drive or read the newspaper, nor could he see the TV clearly.

I explained to him that the bleeding in the right eye was caused by vein occlusion that needed laser treatment to prevent further bleeding, and that I could do the treatment in my office. I understood that transportation was a problem for Slim, so I offered to do the laser treatment on the same visit.

The treatment went well and he was scheduled to have the cataract in his left eye removed in a couple of weeks.

That surgery also went well, and I saw him the next day for follow-up. As usual, Slim said little and didn't seem to be very happy.

"Are you doing alright?" I asked. "Are things going well at the home?"

Slim frowned. "That hell hole is no good for anybody. The food is inedible. The whole place smells like urine, and it's so noisy all the time, with this crazy woman who wails day and night. I don't think I can stand that place any longer," he complained.

"What are your options?" I asked.

"Not many, I guess," he replied with a shrug. "I was told to move to this place because I had a minor stroke, and the cataracts mean I can't drive or read. If I could see better and the weakness in my left leg gets better, maybe I could rent a small apartment and live on my own."

I told him about Mr. Hajibian and how happy he was at the Armenian Home.

"Yeah, I've heard good things about the Armenian Home," Slim nodded. "But I think it's only for Armenians. You know, the Armenians and the Okies didn't get along when both groups first arrived in the Valley. My parents thought the Armenians weren't honest people, and I was told that the Armenians thought us Okies were stupid and uneducated. I don't think the Armenian Home would be good for me."

As I listened to Slim, I was thinking how difficult it must be for a person who has grown old and hasn't been able to save money along the way, with no pension. It must be so sad to be old and poor, I thought.

Slim was pleased that he was already seeing better with the eye that had the cataract surgery, and he said his right eye that had the laser treatment also seemed better.

"If I can drive again, I'll have more options," he remarked.

"Mr. Allred, I'm curious about Twilight Haven. Do you mind if I visit you this Sunday?" I asked.

"I don't understand why you'd want to visit that place," he said. "I think you'll find it depressing. Yes, I'd love to see you there."

Sunday, after church and our regular visit to the donut shop, I told my family that I needed to stop by a nursing home to see a patient, and they could eat the donuts while they waited.

Slim was right that the place reeked of urine. It was noisy, with people crying, moaning and occasionally screaming. I suspected there must be patients with dementia at this home.

Slim shared a room with another man, a man with severe emphysema who was on oxygen. He was very quiet, barely moving. Slim was sitting up in his bed watching TV.

"Hi Doc," he greeted. "I can see the TV clearer now. The colors are brighter now."

"I'm very glad you're seeing better," I said.

As I did a quick examination of his eyes, Slim complained, "I'm so sick and tired of the food here. I was told that because of my high blood pressure and stroke, I have to be on a low-salt, low-fat diet. The canned beans taste terrible. I don't know what kind of fish they serve, but it tastes like rubber. It must've been frozen for a long time.

"Doc, would you do me a favor? A month ago, my niece visited me and I talked her into buying fish and chips for me. Long John Silver's is half a block from here. Please, would you get three pieces and some fries for me? I'm so hungry for some decent food," pleaded Slim.

"Mr. Allred, your doctor put you on such a diet for good reason. I could get into trouble if I got the fish and chips for you. You don't want to have another stroke," I reasoned.

"Doc, at my age, I don't really care," he responded. "What's the point of being alive if you're miserable? It's been over a month since I ate something I liked. Please just do this once. I'll never ask you to do it again," he begged.

"Well, I'll make sure they don't put any salt on your fish and chips," I compromised. "Don't you tell anyone that your eye doctor got it for you," I smiled.

I went out to the car, where the children were getting restless. I'd been inside for almost half an hour and the donuts were long gone.

"I need to run an errand for my patient," I explained. "We need to go by Long John Silver's and get a fish and chips meal for him." I didn't mention that Slim was on a low-salt, low-fat diet.

I rushed into the fish place and got three pieces of halibut and fries to go with them. No salt was added to the fish or fries. I got containers of vinegar and ketchup, and a medium diet Coke.

As soon as I entered his room, Slim got up from his bed and sat in his chair. "Doc, you don't know how much this means to me," he said. "Even if it costs a week of my life, it will be worth it," he declared as he took his first bite of the halibut.

He seemed to enjoy every morsel of the fish, and every bite of the fries, dipping the fish into the vinegar and soaking his fries in ketchup. As he drank the ice cold Coke, he had his eyes closed as if to savor every drop.

Again, I thought how hard it was to be old and poor, without a family.

As I bid Slim goodbye, he smiled and said, "Doc, I'll always remember you for this."

I exited the home and joined my family with a smile on my face, looking like the cat that swallowed the canary.

"What's the smile about?" Mary asked suspiciously. She knew me better and was certain I'd done something naughty. We'd been married too long!

I told her about Slim's diet and how he'd been craving the fish and chips.

"You are a very bad doctor!" Mary exclaimed.

"I know, I am," I responded.

We both laughed.

***

Ojos Verdes...

Consuelo Mendez was referred to me by her ophthalmologist in Merced because of her retinal detachment in the right eye as well as diabetic retinopathy.

She was a quiet woman who looked older than her stated age of 60, her round face etched with wrinkles and her hair tied into a bun at the back. She was stout, about five feet tall, and she had the most beautiful bright green eyes.

Accompanying her was her son, Bobby, who looked exactly like her except that he was much taller and wider. He reminded me somewhat of the comedian Dom DeLuise. He was effeminate and walked and talked with exaggerated hand gestures, much like the stereotypical gay men I'd seen in movies.

Mother and son shared the same round face, bright green eyes and the same tiny nose. But Bobby was loquacious compared to Consuelo, who was reserved and said little.

As Consuelo was my last patient of the day, I had a little extra time to socialize. As I examined her, I remarked on her beautiful green eyes.

"Yes," Bobby said, "when my dad was alive many years ago, he used to call her *mi Ojos Verdes*—my green eyes in Spanish.

When I was young, I thought they were such a cool couple when my father took my mom for a ride on his Harley and sang *Aquellos Ojos Verdes*—Those Green Eyes.

"He was a mechanic and was crazy about motorcycles, but unfortunately he got in an accident one rainy night and was killed," Bobby said sadly. "My poor mom had to work to support us five kids."

Consuelo had a total retinal detachment in her right eye, and from her history I learned that it had happened about a day ago, so the sooner we did the surgery, the better her chances of recovering most of her vision.

I did the surgery that evening, and everything went well. Consuelo stayed in the hospital for one night and was sent home with Bobby the following day.

My parents now lived in Oakland, and it was my custom to visit them about once a month, usually driving up on a Saturday and staying until Sunday afternoon. As it was on my way, I called and told Bobby that I'd make a house call at noon that Saturday, which Bobby said he'd have to miss, since Saturday was usually the busiest day at the flower shop where he worked.

It was a beautiful drive. I followed Bobby's directions and found their house, which was about ten miles east of Merced.

The Valley is full of little towns like Planada. I had read up on this town and found out that Planada was originally named Whitton by railroad officials. The area's first settlers was a group of white Swiss dairy farmers, who renamed the settlement Geneva, and later the town was renamed Planada. Now, most of the residents were Hispanics, with a total population of about 4,000.

The Mendez residence was a small house right along the country road. It was beautifully maintained, with flowers in front and a few citrus trees at the side of the house.

I knocked at the front door and heard footsteps inside, and Consuelo opened the door. She wore a patch over her right eye, which I'd instructed Bobby to change daily.

"How are you feeling?" I asked as she ushered me into the living room.

"Really good," she replied. "It was easier than I thought, and there hasn't been any pain."

I helped her to the couch to sit down and removed the eye patch. Then, standing six feet away with an eye chart, I asked her to read the letters. To my amazement, she was able to read the 20/40 line.

Examination of the retina showed that it was fully reattached and there was no sign of infection or bleeding.

"Doc, I can see clearly and I don't feel any pain," she exclaimed. She got up and headed for the kitchen, returning shortly with a cup of coffee.

"Do you want milk and sugar?" she asked.

"Black is fine for me," I answered, taking the cup from her.

She got her own coffee and sat back down on the couch next to me.

"How long have you lived in Planada?" I asked.

"I've lived in this house for over fifty years," she replied. "My parents left Texas because they heard there were jobs in the area. I was only ten when we arrived. I was actually born in Texas.

"I raised five children in this house," Consuelo continued, "and they're all married except Bobby. Now it's just Bobby and me here."

"Bobby seems like a very good son," I remarked.

"Yes, he is a good boy," she said with a smile. "I don't know what I would do without him. He's saving money so he can buy the flower shop from his boss someday."

"What kind of work did you do to raise your kids?" I asked.

"When my husband died, I had to work," she answered. "I picked fruit. It was really hard work. About ten years ago, I got a job at the De Silva Dairy helping with the cleaning and other chores. It's not as bad as picking fruit and the boss is kind, and I'm provided with health insurance and even a pension."

"That's great," I said, impressed by how hard she'd worked to support her family. "Anything interesting to see in Planada?" I asked.

Consuelo shrugged and said, "It's a one street town with a restaurant and bar and a few small groceries. Most people shop in Merced. There's really nothing going on in this town."

The grandfather clock in her living room struck 1 o'clock. I thanked Consuelo for the coffee and gathered my medical bag.

As she walked me to the door, I said, "Mrs. Mendez, I'm so glad that you're doing well. It's wonderful visiting you and I get a chance to see for myself what Planada is like. Tell Bobby that I'd like to see you again in my office in two or three weeks. If you have any questions or problems, call me."

"Dr. Hung, thank you so much for stopping by," Consuelo said sincerely.

I gave her a hug and headed to my car.

As I continued the drive to Oakland, the sun was shining and most of the fruit trees were in bloom, bursting with white or pink flowers. It was a beautiful sight. It was a wonderful day.

It is so true that *each interaction between a doctor and a patient is a story*. I've learnt so much by asking my patients about their lives. Each person has a distinct story to tell. As a doctor, I believe we should get out of our comfort zone and try to understand the world our patients live in.

Chapter 32
MaryAnne

IN MEDICAL SCHOOL, we were reminded not to treat our own family members except under certain conditions. This is the AMA's position on the issue:

> When the patient is an immediate family member, the physician's personal feelings may unduly influence his or her professional medical judgment. Or the physician may fail to probe sensitive areas when taking the medical history or to perform intimate parts of the physical examination. Physicians may feel obligated to provide care for family members despite feeling uncomfortable doing so. They may also be inclined to treat problems that are beyond their expertise or training.
>
> Similarly, patients may feel uncomfortable receiving care from a family member. A patient may be reluctant to disclose sensitive information or undergo an intimate examination when the physician is an immediate family member. This discomfort may particularly be the case when the patient is a minor child, who may not feel free to refuse care from a parent.
>
> In general, physicians should not treat themselves or members of their own families. However, it may be acceptable to do so in limited circumstances:
>
> (a) In emergency settings or isolated settings where there is no other qualified physician available. In such situations,

Melanoma is a cancer that begins in the melanocytes. Other names for this cancer include malignant melanoma and cutaneous melanoma. Most melanoma cells still make melanin, so melanoma tumors are usually brown or black.

I asked MaryAnne how long she'd had it and she said she didn't know. Mary didn't know either. Since nobody seemed to know how long the lesion had been there, I assumed that it was a fast-growing cancer.

My mind went blank. I was horrified. That evening, I couldn't eat and I was preoccupied, thinking about the lesion.

That night, I barely slept. My mind was racing to figure out how to deal with MaryAnne's "malignant melanoma."

Looking back, now I realize that I was "catastrophizing"—jumping to the worst scenario conclusion. I was certain that she had cancer.

The next morning, I went to the office early and tried to come up with a plan to tackle the problem. I decided that the lesion had to come out as soon as possible.

I called my general surgeon friend, Dr. Newfeld, but he was back in Vancouver visiting his family. I called my plastic surgeon friend, Dr. Gillian, but I was told that he was attending a conference in New York.

My mind was made up that the lesion had to come out that day. I made another call to another general surgeon friend. He said he could see MaryAnne the following Monday, commenting that it was unusual for a child for have melanoma, especially someone who was half Chinese.

By now, I had become irrational. I needed do something for MaryAnne. That lesion had to come out. I called Dr. Carl Chen, the best pathologist in the Valley, who had published countless articles and was well-known in the country. Dr. Chen owed me a big favor after I'd helped his parents out when they came from Taiwan a few years earlier. Both had multiple eye problems of glaucoma and cataract. They were Hakka like me, so they felt at home because I could speak to them in their dialect. I did surgery on both of them, and both had great results and were very pleased.

I told Dr. Chen the situation and asked him if he would do a frozen section of MaryAnne's lesion, which I was going to remove. He was more than happy to return me a favor and said that one of his assistants in the lab would come by my office with some bottles and wait to take the specimen back to him. He'd be able to tell me from the frozen section if the lesion was cancerous or not within half an hour.

I called Mary and told her to bring MaryAnne into the office. With the help of my assistant Monta, I anesthetized the area on MaryAnne's leg. I had marked off the lesion, leaving a wide margin to make sure I got all the growth. I carefully dissected around the lesion, noting that the underlying tissue seemed normal, and just the skin was involved.

The entire lesion with a wide margin was removed and placed in the bottle that Dr. Chen's assistant had brought, and she promptly left to take the specimen for Dr. Chen to examine. I then carefully closed the wound with medium-sized black silk sutures, meticulously re-approximating the wound.

As I waited for the results of the frozen section, feeling desperate, I had a conversation with myself, saying I would give up all my wealth and all my education for MaryAnne to be free of cancer.

Half an hour later, Dr. Chen called. The lesion was not cancerous. It was a hemangioma, a tumor of the blood vessels, and the margin was free of any such cells. I'd done a clean excision of the growth.

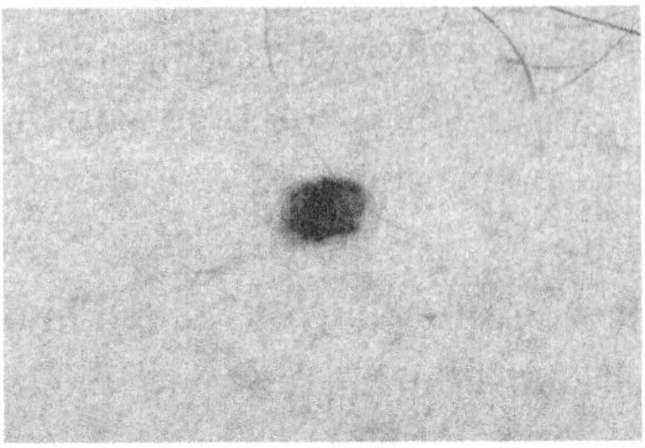

A hemangioma

Hemangiomas of the skin develop when there's an abnormal proliferation of blood vessels in one area of the body. Experts aren't sure why blood vessels group together like this.

Dr. Chen said it was an unusual presentation of hemangioma because it was darker than most. But he was sure that it wasn't cancerous, and the regular slides would give him more details on the kind of cells involved. He would have the full pathology report ready by Monday.

I was tremendously relieved that my daughter didn't have cancer; but, perhaps because of all the tension of the last 24 hours, my mind would not shut down. For the rest of the day I was still preoccupied with the lesion. I tried to understand how I got myself so worked up and convinced that it was melanoma.

A week later, I tried to remove the sutures. The wound was still sensitive, and MaryAnne, who was now ten, had strong legs. She kicked and tried to stop me, but with Mary's help I managed to remove them.

In addition to doing surgery on people's eyes, I also did surgery on people's eyelids and faces for many years. As a rule, we usually removed the sutures in a week or so, to minimize scar formation. I'd forgotten that the thigh is much more muscular and the skin much tougher. Because I'd removed the lesion with a wide margin, there was tension in the wound. As soon as I removed the last suture, MaryAnne's wound broke open.

By then, I was so upset with myself that I asked Mary to take MaryAnne to see the plastic surgeon about what to do next.

Dr. Gillian, my plastic surgeon friend, examined MaryAnne's leg and recommended doing nothing, as the wound would heal by granulation.

It was a big lesson for me. I still couldn't understand how I'd worked myself into an almost irrational state. The truth of the matter was that the lesion didn't have to be removed that day. It could have waited until one of the surgeons was available.

In addition, although removing the lesion was well within my expertise, I made the mistake of removing the sutures too early.

Now, I firmly believe in not treating one's family members. You can no longer be objective when a loved one is involved.

In the end, this story had a happy ending. The scar was barely noticeable and MaryAnne forgave me.

Made in the USA
Monee, IL
04 November 2026

67386429R10174